The Bad Acts
of the Apostles

John Henson

First published by O Books, 2009
O Books is an imprint of John Hunt Publishing Ltd., The Bothy, Deershot Lodge, Park Lane, Ropley,
Hants, SO24 0BE, UK
office1@o-books.net
www.o-books.net

Distribution in:

UK and Europe
Orca Book Services
orders@orcabookservices.co.uk
Tel: 01202 665432 Fax: 01202 666219Int. code
(44)

USA and Canada
NBN
custserv@nbnbooks.com
Tel: 1 800 462 6420 Fax: 1 800 338 4550

Australia and New Zealand
Brumby Books
sales@brumbybooks.com.au
Tel: 61 3 9761 5535 Fax: 61 3 9761 7095

Far East (offices in Singapore, Thailand, Hong
Kong, Taiwan)
Pansing Distribution Pte Ltd
kemal@pansing.com
Tel: 65 6319 9939 Fax: 65 6462 5761

South Africa
Alternative Books
altbook@peterhyde.co.za
Tel: 021 555 4027 Fax: 021 447 1430

Text copyright John Henson 2008

Design: Stuart Davies

ISBN: 978 1 84694 169 6

A CIP catalogue record for this book is available
from the British Library.

Printed by CPI Antony Rowe, Chippenham and Eastbourne

O Books operates a distinctive and ethical publishing philosophy in
all areas of its business, from its global network of authors to
production and worldwide distribution.
This book is produced on FSC certified stock, within ISO14001
standards. The printer plants sufficient trees each year through
the Woodland Trust to absorb the level of emitted carbon in
its production.

The Bad Acts of the Apostles

John Henson

BOOKS

Winchester, UK
Washington, USA

This work is dedicated to
Rowan Williams, Archbishop of Canterbury,
From a grateful recipient of his friendship.

CONTENTS

Foreword

You hold in your hand a book crafted by John Henson. You may not yet be aware of the danger that lies before you.

My first significant encounter with John Henson took place on the Southern coast of Wales. Since I was a foreign visitor to John's Welsh homeland, he acted as the good host and offered to take me to a nearby beach. I have been to many different beaches before - in North America, South America, Southern Europe and the Caribbean. I thought I knew what to expect, and since John alluded to nothing out of the ordinary, I innocently let him lead me to his favorite beach. From the car park we walked down a narrow muddy lane, over a pile of stones, between several tall hedges, through a gate, and eventually down a hill and around a corner. I froze.

A wall of Rock towered above the shoreline. Giant flat stones like ancient paving from a colossal cathedral long ago lost to the sea stretched out before us. The sun shone brightly on the waves as they pounded these stones. Guided by John, I crossed over the magnificent hard surface until my bare feet landed in soft, smooth sand. Both imposing and inviting, this beach confronted me with a bold new construct of what a beach could be.

But even more imposing and inviting than this wild, whimsical Welsh shoreline, John Henson, with his razor sharp intellect and breathtakingly fresh insights captured my mind and heart. We talked all that afternoon under a clear sunny sky and discussed scripture, church history, sexuality, family, politics, mental illness, gardening and Jesus. I marveled to discover a man so brilliant and well-educated with such a tender heart and delicate disposition. That one day on that one beach with John Henson and our diverse channels of conversation stimulated and fed me for many months. The memory still nourishes me today.

John Henson causes people to think in new directions, to

consider divergent views, and to feel afresh the impact of the Good News of Jesus. And this creates problems! For once his revolutionary insights and deliciously subversive words enter our minds, they demand a response. No simple academic comprehension will do.

If you wish to remain unruffled in your view of the world, of scripture and of yourself, I STRONGLY RECOMMEND that you immediately put down The Bad Acts of the Apostles.

But if you would embrace an adventure of thought, feeling and imagination, then like I did that fine summer day on the Southern coast of Wales, I urge you to run towards the crashing waves and dive right in. But remember, you have been warned.

Peterson Toscano, a theatrical performance activist, a Quaker and a vegan, travels throughout North America and Europe stirring up trouble and thought with his one-person comedies.

Introduction

It was the second time I had climbed to the top of Pen-Y-Fan. I took with me two visitors to Wales. On the previous occasion I had been shown the way by another friend. Pen-Y-Fan is the highest mountain in South Wales, and from its height there is a glorious view encompassing all the counties of Wales as well as several counties of England. On a good day, Yr Wyddfa (Snowdon), the highest peak in all Wales, can be seen. From the top of Pen-Y-Fan run several rivulets that together merge, south of the mountain, to form the river Taf. As great a thrill as the view from the top, on the occasion of my first climb, was to drink the water direct from the spring that led to one of these streams. The taste was like to the nectar of the gods. I was relating this experience to my companions on my second visit as we started from the mountain pass at the bottom to follow the main stream upwards. It was a hot day and very nearly were we enticed to cup our hands in the stream and taste the waters that ran so close to their source. It was as well we did not, for just a few yards yonder we saw lying right across the stream the rotting carcass of a dead sheep attended by a coterie of dung flies. All the water below that level was being filtered through that grizzly lump of putrefaction.

The Acts of the Apostles was written by Luke, the author of the Gospel. As it appears in the Christian scriptures, Acts forms a kind of sequel to the Gospel, as Luke's reference at its beginning to 'my first book' seems to indicate. The traditional title, 'The Acts of the Apostles' is somewhat misleading, since only a few of the apostles get a look in. 'Glimpses into the life of some of the very first Christians' might serve as a title for the first part of the work; 'The missionary journeys of Paul' for the second half. Some see Acts as a description of the continuation of the ministry of Jesus through the Spirit. In the light of my experience on Pen-Y-Fan I would urge caution. To provide some kind of record of the

1

earliest years of the first Christian communities was doubtless one of Luke's motives. But this was probably second to his purpose of extolling the merits of his hero and mentor Paul, a controversial and far from universally loved figure at the time. To show the work of Paul to be equal to that of Rocky (Peter) was possibly the reason why the activities of Rocky are so well covered in the first part, so that Luke can draw very clear parallels between the careers of the two pioneers. Both escape from prison; both heal a disabled man; both bring someone back from the point of death; both convert a Roman officer – and so on. The other consideration that makes it misleading to regard Acts as a sequel to the Gospel is that the two works as we have them were probably not written in sequence. Scholars generally believe that Luke's Gospel began as a shorter work including some of the material peculiar to Luke, some similar to that contained in Matthew, and some similar to that found in Mark. Luke then proceeded to write Acts. Sometime later the whole of Mark's Gospel became available to him and he folded this additional material into his own gospel, only omitting where he already had material dealing with the same events. Thus instead of thinking of Luke as writing the Gospel and Acts in sequence, we must rather think of him as going from one to the other and back again, perhaps re-ordering and editing more than once. This is the way many of the great composers, including Beethoven, wrote their symphonies. This gave Luke, the highly competent author and shrewd thinker, opportunity to reflect on the correspondence between the work of Jesus and the subsequent progress of the Church. With such a wealth of material on the conduct and teachings of Jesus available to him, it would indeed be very surprising if Luke never asked the question, "How are the followers of Jesus measuring up to their teacher?"

Until now Christians have always assumed that Luke's purpose was to congratulate the 'apostles' on how well they were doing in being faithful to the intentions of Jesus, and to set forth a blueprint for the life of the Christian community for all time. The more I read Acts, the more I become convinced that this is not the case. Luke does recount many of the stories in Acts in accents of admiration and with a view to inspiring later generations. His account of the death of Steven leaps quickly to mind. But I have also come to notice that Luke sometimes seems to record events dispassionately, and in the case of others I detect veiled criticism. I feel sure that if the activities of the first Christians contrasted unfavourably with what he was noting down about the life and teachings of Jesus at the time, he would not approve, though it might not suit his purposes to criticise the church leaders too obviously since they were having a hard time of it striving to achieve some measure of discipline and combating emerging heresies. There are more than a few occasions recorded in Acts where the apostles deviated seriously from the clear intentions of Jesus. These Luke must surely have noticed and thus recorded them not in order to provide an example for us to follow, but as a warning as to how quickly a religious movement can be polluted, and how close to its source. There are other events that Luke recorded, about which he may not have come to such a severe judgement, but which we with hindsight and reflection may disapprove because we can see where they depart from Jesus, even if Luke could not. The fact that Luke has provided the evidence, however, makes him a party to our findings.

This rather different approach to Acts has some serious implications. There are Christians who pride themselves on being 'apostolic'. Their faith is founded foursquare on that of the apostles. Others have deviated! If, however, the apostles themselves deviated seriously in some respects from the intentions of Jesus, and if, to some extent, it was the purpose of Luke to demonstrate this, then being 'apostolic' or in an 'apostolic succession' is no great shakes! Paul converted Luke, and it was Paul who wrote, **'The bricklayer must be careful to build up from the foundation already in place. No one should try to replace it with another. The foundation is Jesus, God's Chosen.'**

3

(Paul's first letter to Corinth 3:11.) This follows on from a passage in which Paul specifically warns of the dangers of founding the Church on its first leaders. **'What's so big about Ray or Paul? We're only helpers, doing the job God has given us. I put the plants in the pots, and Ray came along with the watering can. It was God who got the plants to grow. The one who pots and the one who waters, are nothing compared with the gardener who produces the plants.'**(Ray = Apollos, after 'Apollo' the sun god.)

Although it is far from easy to trace the stream back to its pure source in Jesus, since the documents we possess were written by disciples or disciples of disciples, we can never be satisfied with a Christianity that behaves in ways Jesus would not approve. Only when the actions of Rocky and Paul and the other apostles are true to the example set by their Leader, should we strive to imitate them. If they fail to display the mind of Jesus, we must, as Jesus did, tell them to 'get out of our sight'. (Matthew 16: 23 NIV)

Chapter One

"DO IT NOW, LORD!"

'At a time when they were all together, the helpers asked Jesus, "Leader, are you now going to give political power back to the Jewish people?" Jesus said, "The future course of the world's history is none of your business! It's a matter for the Loving God. Your job, when God's Spirit gives you confidence, will be to stand up for me in Jerusalem and the surrounding district, in Samaria and all over the world." Soon after Jesus said this, the friends watched him go up the mountain and disappear among the clouds. As they were straining to get a last look at Jesus going on his way, a couple of people wearing bright clothes came up to them and said, "What are you folk from Galilee looking up there for? You've only lost sight of Jesus for a while. He'll come back the way he went, and he'll still be the same Jesus!"Luke Part Two (Acts) 1:6.

Jesus said, "If the leaders of your community tell you God's New World is in the sky, you'll know they've got it wrong. That's where the birds will discover the New World! To say the New World is in the sky is as silly as saying it's under the sea. That's where the fish will discover it! In fact, God's New World has no precise location. It's to be found inside you and all around you." Thought-Provoking Sayings (Gospel of Thomas) chapter 1.

The very first example of criticism by Luke of the apostles is clearly so. Is he perhaps introducing a theme for much that is to follow? Before Jesus parts from his friends for the last time, they pose the question, "Leader, are you now going to give political power back to the Jewish people?" Nothing could be more damning than this question as an indication of how little the disciples of Jesus had paid attention to their lessons. Jesus had just spent three years trying to explain that 'God's New World' (The Kingdom) is not to

5

be understood as it was popularly understood at that time, in terms of military might and political authority. Jesus had sorted things out in his own mind at the beginning of his ministry in the soul-searching experience in the desert, as Luke knew. That experience set Jesus on a train of thought that enabled him later to assure his followers that it is useless to speculate when or where God's New World will come about, for this New World is already "among you" or "inside you". (The Greek can mean either and probably means both.) When they persisted in arguing about who should be considered the greatest among them, Jesus did not just counsel humility but ruled against aspirations of power based on the example of successful earthly monarchs. (Luke 22: 24-26) Jesus' special helpers (apostles), at his physical parting from them, still did not grasp the idea that God's Chosen (Messiah) and, by implication, his community, were to govern themselves according to the pattern of the 'Servant' described by the prophet of Babylon in the Hebrew scriptures. (Luke 18: 31-34) The way the disciples put their question, the whole tone and feel of it, suggests that it was some kind of obvious triumph they were after. They also assumed that this triumph was to be for the exclusive enjoyment of their own nation. Jesus had sought to teach them otherwise. "People will come down the wide roads from every part of the world to be at the big party to celebrate God's New World. Those now thought of as no-hopers will have the best seats, whereas those who think they deserve special status will be lucky to get a seat at all." (Luke 13:29)

Three hours would probably have not been enough for Jesus to put the disciples right if they had failed to get the message in three years. Luke's opinion we have no need to guess at. After all, he was Greek. He simply records the curt and dismissive reply of Jesus, "The future course of the world's history is none of your business! It is a matter for the Loving God." The question of the apostles was out of order. It always is, even when we substitute, "we, the true and faithful Christians" for Israel. Luke then pointedly records the prediction of Jesus that his friends will

6

promote his cause to every part of the world. There is more to God's New World than Israel, or 'New Israel'.

The question about God's New World must have seemed to Luke more than an innocent enquiry about dates. The question was insidious. It was set to undermine the very basis of the ministry of Jesus. That ministry had begun, according to Luke, with a sermon in which Jesus had used the prophet of Babylon (Isaiah 61) as his manifesto.

> *"God's Spirit has inspired me*
> *to bring the poor good news;*
> *She tells me, 'Get the blind to see,*
> *Bust the jails and set folk free;*
> *God's arms are open lovingly.' "*
> (Luke 4: 16-21)

Nothing could be further from this manifesto than the triumphant political vindication of Israel implied by the disciples' question. Jesus had proceeded in that sermon to cite from the pages of history the single mother of Lebanon and Norman the Syrian leper as examples of God's grace to people of other lands, for which extremity Jesus was nearly thrown over a cliff top. It is not credible that Luke, of all people, could fail to notice the difference between the commencement of the ministry of Jesus and that of his disciples. Jesus proclaimed a universal new society based on justice and compassion. His disciples were reverting to a narrow and vindictive nationalism. The first heresy was the heresy of 'Triumphalism' rampant in so many of the choruses sung nowadays. The originators of this heresy were the apostles!

I want to tell you now about my one and only visit to Bury St. Edmunds. It was one of those rare single occasions in my life that have affected my theology. I visited a holy place and came back having progressed, I trust, in my understanding of God. I hope St.

Edmund is pleased.

It was a Spring Bank holiday and I was staying with a friend of mine in the Baptist ministry in north London. We decided to avoid a day out in London and to make instead for the fresh air and green fields of Suffolk. We got into the car without any clear plan of where we were going and arrived about lunchtime at Bury St. Edmunds, somewhere I had never been before, nor my friend either, I think. We parked in a street car park just opposite the entrance to the ruins of the old abbey. We had just locked the car door and were about to cross the road for the abbey when around the corner to our right came the beginnings of what was to prove a long procession. They were people of all ages, many of them young, divided into succeeding groups with banners. The first banner announced to us that these were the Baptists of Suffolk making for a venue where they were to hold a rally. The other banners had been made to identify the various individual churches or groups represented. My friend suggested that we position ourselves behind the car since he could already see one or two faces he recognized. Since our purpose on that Bank holiday was to have a day off, he did not want us to be drawn into the event. The number of Baptists mustered for the occasion was impressive. The procession went on and on. But I was not impressed by the nature of this Christian act of witness. I became more and more agitated as the procession progressed. There were many other on-lookers, but nothing in the procession attracted us to it. The marchers hardly looked at us, so there was no need to hide behind the car. They were noticeably self-absorbed. Nobody shouted 'hello' or 'good morning' to us or 'God bless you in the name of Jesus'. Nobody was handing out leaflets. Most of the onlookers, unlike ourselves, did not even have the advantage of knowing what a Baptist was. The marchers were singing songs of triumph from their chorus books. One I recognized has the oft-repeated phrase, "Our God Reigns". It comes from a good Advent song, but it is a pity the songwriter so frequently uses the phrase "Our God Reigns", since the original scripture text is "Your God Reigns". The inclusive invitation of the Hebrew prophet is thus twisted to serve as watchword of an exclusive and possessive Church. The enthusiastic songsters sounded just like the supporters of a winning football team. "We are the Champions." Whatever their intentions, to the outside observer, as I was that day, these people seemed out to show us how many there were of them. Like marches of a more political nature, it was a demonstration of strength by numbers. Sorry, Baptists of Suffolk, I could not applaud you as you passed along, though I'm sure you are good people and love Jesus. I simply describe truthfully how I felt that day.

The procession at last over, we were able to cross the road and visit the abbey ruins. These are extensive but I'm never very impressed by ruins and besides we have so many splendid ruins to choose from in my native land of Wales. However, something memorable happened while we were sitting in a small enclosure facing an attractive flowerbed, eating our packed lunch. We were visited by a blackbird. We quickly noticed there was something wrong with him. He had injured one of his wings in some way and was unable to fly. He fluttered helplessly around the garden, not able to get himself more than a foot off the ground. Then suddenly he stopped quite near us and looked at us. He then opened his mouth and forth came the full flow of his beautiful blackbird song. It was a spine chilling experience. He seemed to be saying. Alright, you've noticed, I can't fly, but I can still sing. He seemed to me to be saying something about the Resurrection, about life from the dead, about the strength that is born out of weakness. Any time he might be caught by a cat. He was so vulnerable. His was not the strength in numbers claimed by the marchers. But I found his song much sweeter.

After we had rested we made for the large church beside the abbey ruins. It was one of three churches that had originally been attached to the abbey, two only surviving. This large one had become the Cathedral. We had a look around the cathedral, which was just a large church converted for the purpose. One thing puzzled us. Everywhere the church or town was mentioned on a notice board, it was not Bury St. Edmunds, but St. Edmundsbury. As we were going out we decided to ask the verger at the door if he could offer an explanation. "Ah", he said, "that's a very important distinction. St. Edmondsbury is the correct name for the town. In the old days, when the town was an important religious centre and a place of pilgrimage, the abbey ruled the town. The church imposed lots of restrictions on town life and levied taxes. When under Henry VIII the abbey was abolished the people of the town and district were very pleased about it and jokingly said, 'We're going to bury St. Edmunds!' The name stuck." Then a big grin came over the verger's face and he said, "But, you see, we've won! Our abbey church has become a cathedral and you see the bishop's chair up the front. And a wealthy American is going to pay for us to have a spire so that everyone can see we've a cathedral for miles around. WE'VE WON!"

For the second time of the day I felt very uncomfortable and that I did not have a lot in common with my fellow-Christian. "We've won!" Is that what it's about? "Our God reigns!" It wasn't difficult, as a history graduate, with the Tudor period my favourite, to imagine what an oppressive presence the abbey church had been to the people of that town. What an indictment that they were glad to see the abbey disappear and much of it reduced to ruins. What an indictment that church and townsfolk were such bitter rivals, and rivals still, it would seem. How sorry I was, when I thought about it, that the verger did not tell me what the cathedral was doing for the community in the name of Jesus. Were there homeless in Bury St. Edmunds? If so, was the church doing anything to help? What was it doing for young people? What for the elderly? What for those needing counseling and befriending? More than likely something was being done and still being done. But all the verger could tell me was, "We've won!"

Very early in the history of the Christian Church the event of the Ascension became linked to some of the psalms in the Hebrew Scriptures. These psalms are known as "Psalms of Ascent". They celebrate the annual procession of the Ark of the Covenant to Jerusalem. The King of Glory comes to his throne. There he sits in state and triumphs over his enemies. The enemies are, of course, foreign foes, enemies of the state. The procession and ritual enthroning of God, very like that of an eastern potentate, was an exercise in self-confidence for the team.

This is the line the church has taken down the ages when it celebrates the Ascension. Jesus, the King of Glory, is going up in triumph to his eternal throne. There he reigns for ever and ever, ensuring victory for his people.

'He sits at God's right hand till all his foes submit,
And bow at his command, and fall beneath his feet."

Is this what Jesus had in mind when he said, "Those who humble themselves will be exalted."; "the first shall be last and the last shall be first"; "the one who wishes to be great among you must be the everybody's slave." ?? When we sing hymns and choruses about power and majesty and dominion and authority, do we have the same mindset as the one whose throne was a cross, and who wore a crown of thorns? Are we in line with the one whose arms stretch out to embrace not the few, but all? The one who does not boast of success like St. Edmund's verger, but sings in his weakness like St. Edmund's blackbird.

Jesus Comes

(1) Jesus comes with streamers flying,
Once as friend of outcasts killed;
Crowds of keen supporters with him,
Mouths with joyful laughter filled:
Loudly cheering (x3)
Ears and eyes and hearts are thrilled.

(2) There's no mistaking this time round;
Perfect love now understood;
We who spat and sent him bound,
Broken, to a cross of wood,
Truly sorry (x3)
Glad that wrath is not his mood.

(3) Dare we look or shyly glance
At that body full of grace?
Marks of thorns and nails and lance,
Sorrow lingering on his face?
Brightly smiling! (x3)
All our anxious fears give place.

4) Humble Jesus, same as ever,
Spurns a throne of grand design;
Loving always, judging never;
Towel and basin still the sign;
You will be with us (x3)
When we greet the end of time.

(5) Merriment and quiet worship
Mingle as we work and wait;
For it is no tyrant lordship
We with dread anticipate;
Ours is the hurry (x3)
He'll be not a moment late.

(After Charles Wesley. Tune: Helmsley.)

Chapter Two

WHY ARE WE WAITING?

On one occasion, there were about a hundred and twenty people in the room. Rocky stood up to make a speech. He said, "Friends, you can't stop the Old Books coming true. God's Spirit spoke through David and foresaw that Judas would help to get Jesus arrested. Judas was one of us and assisted us in God's work." (You may like to know what happened to Judas. He bought a field with the money he was given for betraying Jesus. He had a bad fall there and was fatally injured. When the people of Jerusalem got to hear about it, they called his field "The Bloody Field".)Rocky went on, "One of our songs goes like this,

> *'His house will be empty,*
> *Its owner gone:*
> *And his job will be going too...'*

We need a replacement to join us in the job of convincing people Jesus is alive. It must be someone who belonged to our group all the time Jesus our Leader shared his life with us, from the time John was dipping in the river, to the day Jesus went out of our sight up the mountain." There were two candidates, Joseph (sometimes known as 'Honest Joe') and Matt. Then they spoke to God like this, "God, you know what each of us is really like inside. Show us who you'd like to have in this special job, which Judas gave up to go his own way." Then they put the names in a bag and Matt's name was picked out. He joined the other eleven friends of Jesus with special duties.Luke Part Two (Acts) 1: 15-26.

According to Luke, when Jesus addressed his followers for the last time, he included one clear, unmistakable instruction.

"Don't go away from Jerusalem. Wait till you get what my Parent means to give you. I've talked about it before. John dipped people in water, but in a matter of days you'll be drenched with God's Spirit." (Luke Part 2:4)

Dutifully they returned to Jerusalem and to the room that was their headquarters, possibly the 'Upper Room' where they had shared a special meal with Jesus on his betrayal night. That was the easy bit. But wait for the Spirit's guidance they did not. **Rocky stood up to make a speech.** This agrees with the character of Rocky as we know it from the gospels, including Luke. "Leader, I'm ready to go to prison with you, and to die by your side!" (22:33) Hasty and ill considered words- we know the sequel. Rocky was an impatient man. He seems to have lacked the ability to contemplate at any length, or to weigh his words. Inaction was a torment to him. Instead of waiting for the promised guidance of God's Spirit, he proposed there and then to have an election for the vacancy caused by the defection and death of Judas. Were it not for the advice of Jesus to wait, the idea would seem a sensible one. There had been a breach in their ranks. It is not bad to use a lull in activity to repair defences, to polish up the organization and to prepare for the next stage. It is possible, however, to view the outcome as a mistake. In view of Luke's championship of Paul in the second half of 2Luke, there is more than a hint as to who Luke thought should be the twelfth apostle. But at the time of the election Paul had not even been converted. Precisely! Considerations of issues without the guidance of the Spirit is equivalent to confining the discussion within known categories. The demands of the Gentile mission, for example, could not at this stage be guessed at, nor the sort of qualifications that would be required.

The disciples in the Upper Room were right in turning to prayer and in studying the scriptures. But without opening the window of imagination the Spirit provides, prayer is likely to be directed towards fixed and rigid requests, and the interpretation of scripture will be prejudiced. The prayer had to do with 'which candidate?' rather than 'should we be doing this at all?' The interpretation of scripture is lurid. Rocky chose to expound for the occasion two of the most vindictive psalms – 69 and 109 – which call for vengeance upon the enemy. There was nothing unusual about the literalist picking of texts out of context. Jesus had done the same, though with a unique sensitivity as to the original meaning. (For example, he understood that the story of Sodom had to do with a breach of hospitality.) What is at issue is not Rocky's use of texts in a time-honored way, but his choice of texts and the lack of the spirit of Jesus the choice displayed. The teaching of Jesus that we should love our enemies (1Luke 6: 27) made it inappropriate to choose texts expressing hatred to enemies to make a point. The psalm that Jesus chose to express his feelings about Judas- Psalm 41- expresses sorrow at the betrayal of a friend and depression caused by the attacks of enemies, but is notable in that it contains not the slightest hint of vindictiveness. Rocky chose his psalms because of the way he was feeling, and the way he was feeling meant he was not in a fit state to make decisions or guide others as to the mind of Jesus. If for no other reason, Rocky should have obeyed the Leader's command to wait, in order to let his poisonous, and in view of his own record, hypocritical feelings towards Judas subside. Love for your enemies is the hardest of Christian exercises and we must not be too down on Rocky on that score. But to turn the heat on someone else (who is not there to reply), in order to cover up your own weaknesses, is a particularly nasty way of behaving, though by no means uncommon. 'Those who have most to hide shout loudest.' It is difficult to absolve Rocky from such behavior, and Luke is not sparing with the evidence.

Perhaps a minor matter, but worth commenting on, is the method these first Christians used to choose the new apostle. They drew lots. It is significant that not even the most enthusiastic claimants of strict apostolic practice use this method of making decisions (it would speed up the process of choosing a new Pope, wouldn't it?).The apostles' method of reaching a decision on this occasion (we do not hear of it again) is a symptom of the lack of confidence that what they were doing was right in the first place. How it operated we do not know. Perhaps the disciples reverted to the use of 'Urim and Thummim', as per the ancient Israelite priests. These may have been two stones, one for 'yes' and one for 'no', placed in a bag, which was then asked the appropriate questions. Needless to say (Luke did not need to say it), there is no reference to any such practice when Jesus chose his friends. (1Luke 6:12)

We cannot help feeling sorry for Matt. It was not his fault he was put upon in the way he was. A lucky escape for 'Honest Jo', too! We do not hear of them ever again, like some of the chapel deacons I recall being chosen too hastily to make up the numbers. However, for all we know, they may have been true and life-long friends of Jesus. Was Paul intended by the Spirit to be the twelfth apostle? Luke probably thought so. Perhaps it should have been Maggie, traditionally known as Mary Magdala, which may mean 'Mary the Magnificent' or 'Mary the Great', since a place called 'Magdala' has never been located. Maggie was the first witness of the Resurrection. To be a witness of the Resurrection was regarded as the prime qualification for apostleship. In the words of Robert Runcie, Archbishop of Canterbury, seeking to convince his timorous Church of the scriptural basis for women priests, she was 'the Apostle to the apostles'. Luke pointedly mentions that the women were present on this occasion, 'praying' (presumably out loud, since silent prayer was a resource not yet developed). They were in the same room as the men, not excluded or sectioned off as in the synagogues, the worship places familiar to them. If only the disciples had waited for the Spirit, the prejudice against a woman apostle would have been overcome. Paul performed his vital work with or without his apostolic hat. (He reckoned he had one!) Maggie performed her important work too, with or without the title of apostle. A salutary reminder of the irrelevance of ecclesiastical appointments! Christians get so worked up about who will be the next Archbishop; so do the media; so do Ladbrokes – an interesting link with the apostolic world! The Spirit always has an alternative scale of priorities, based on a wider vision. Remember Francis of Assisi, and Julian of Norwich, and George Fox and William Booth?

The worst aspect of this incident from 'The Bad Acts of the Apostles' is the motivation revealed in the mind of Rocky and presumably in the minds of at least some of the others. It was a ritual to exorcise the ghost of Judas more than anything else. The passage makes very difficult reading in the context of a Christian service of worship. It is 'X' certificate – it is so un-Christian. Did Luke mean it to strike us in this way? His second book begins with the apostles displaying a vindictive nationalism, which we can be sure that, as an internationalist, Luke did not approve. The apostles follow this almost immediately with a vindictive act against the memory of a man loved by Jesus, but hated by them in that he represented their own betrayal. Luke can hardly have approved of that either. It is not a very promising picture he paints of the beginnings of the Christian Church!

Come, Leader dear

(1) Come, Leader dear, and make your home
In every open mind and heart;
We seek your joy and peace to know
And in your New World play our part.

(2) We need imagination's key,
The human touch, the lover's zeal;
Then we the contours of your love
Will know, though tongue can never tell.

(3) Now may the God whose love extends
Beyond the grasp of any mind,
Be known in beauty recognized
In every type of humankind.

(After Isaac Watts 'Come dearest Lord...' v 3 may be used on its own as a parting 'blessing'.

Chapter Three

PENTECOST SERMON

This was the cue for Rocky to stand up where he could be seen, with the other eleven special friends around him. He shouted to the crowd, "My own people, and everyone here in Jerusalem, if you listen carefully, I'll explain what's going on. We haven't been drinking; it's only nine in the morning! What Joel said in his book is coming true:

One day,' says God, 'I will fill every living thing in a special way. My Spirit will move your children to speak for me; she will excite teenagers with new ideas and give old people dreams about the future. Even those who have no rights, my favorites, will be full of me and speak my words.There will be earth-shattering events. The sun will be eclipsed and the moon appear red, as signs of God's coming among us. Then anyone who acknowledges God will be healed.'

My people, listen to me: I'm going to tell you about Jesus from Nazareth, someone you remember being impressed by, because God did great things through him, proving he was God's agent. He fell into your hands. God knew that was going to happen and made plans. You used foreigners to kill Jesus by hanging him on a cross. But God knew that was going to happen and made plans. You used the Romans to kill Jesus, by hanging him on a cross. But God brought him back to life forever. Death couldn't hold him down. One of the songs David sang has words which could be Jesus talking:

> **'God, I follow you,**
> **You're with me all the time;**
> **Nothing breaks my back,**

Always feeling fine.
Sing a song of joy;
Future holds no fears;
You will not let me rot,
Nor give my loved-ones tears.
You've told me what life's all about:
With you I'll always sing and shout.'

Brothers and sisters, it's not very likely our hero David was talking about himself. He's dead and buried; you can go and see his grave any time you want. He was looking into the future and remembering the promise God had given him, that one of his descendants would carry on where he had left off. David foresaw God's Chosen would come back to life after being dead. That's what he meant by the words,

> **'You will not leave me dead,**
> **or let your Chosen rot.'**

Jesus is the one he was talking about. God brought Jesus back to life, and everyone of us here can swear to the truth of it. He has been granted the highest honor by God his Parent, and God has given him the promised Spirit to pass on to us. That's the explanation of what you're seeing and hearing today! David didn't become one with God in this way, but he said,

> **'God said to my Leader Sit by me,**
> **Then you'll have no enemy.**

So now you all know the truth. Jesus, the one you hung on a cross, God has marked out as the Chosen Leader."

When the people heard this they were deeply shocked and said to Rocky and the others "Friends, what can we do about it?" Rocky said, "You can all turn over a new leaf and be dipped in the name of Jesus the Chosen.

*All the wrong things you've done will be forgiven, and you'll have the gift of God's Spirit. She is promised to you and your families, including those who live a long way away. God's invitation is for everybody. Rocky went on speaking to them and appealing to them, saying things like, "The society we live in is rotten to the core. It's time to take a stand and be different!" All those who took notice of what Rocky was saying were dipped, and the number of Jesus' followers was increased by about three thousand.'*2Luke 2:14-42.

'On Sunday evening, when the friends of Jesus met, they locked the doors of the house, because they were afraid of the police. Jesus joined them and said, "Keep calm everybody!" Then Jesus showed them his hands and his side. The friends went wild with joy when they realized their Leader was alive. Jesus had to say again, "Keep calm! The Loving God gave me a job to do, and now I'm going to give **you** *something to do." They felt the breath of Jesus on them as he said, "Let God's Spirit in! From now on it's your job to free people from their guilt. Otherwise they will remain prisoners of their past mistakes."*Sources Close to Jesus (John's Gospel) 20: 19-23.

Fundamentalists have various ways of coping with passages in the Bible that contradict one another in the matter of reported facts. One way is to clobber the differing versions together and try like Cinderella's sisters to squeeze into a slipper that which just will not go. Either Judas hanged himself, or he fell over in a rocky place and disemboweled himself – you can take your pick. The idea that Judas hung himself and the rope broke so that he disemboweled himself is ludicrous and dishonest. The other method fundamentalists use to prevent awkward questions arising in the minds of the innocent is to direct their attention to one account and to keep quiet about the existence of another. David killed Goliath. It's too good a story to have doubts about! Elsewhere it is stated that someone called Elhanan killed Goliath. (2Samuel 21:19) But there's no need to tell anybody that. They are unlikely to discover it unless their Bible reading is very thorough. If they do, then method 'A' will have to be used. They will be told that Elhanan is an alternative name for David – most unlikely, but they will probably swallow it. It is method 'B' which is usually adopted to prevent anyone realizing that there are alternative, contradictory and irreconcilable versions of the gift of the Spirit to the followers of Jesus. Nearly every Christian knows that the Spirit was given on the Day of Pentecost with a rushing mighty wind and tongues of fire. No encouragement is given from fundamentalists, or indeed from Christian mentors of gentler persuasion who are anxious not to confuse their flocks, to take any notice of the clear account in John's Gospel of the giving of the Spirit by Jesus himself on the day of his Resurrection. The best way of coping with this embarrassing contradiction of Luke's account is to pretend it doesn't exist, especially since there are difficult verses that seem, in the older translations, to bear out High Church ideas about authority.

If we treat the scriptures with more respect, then we shall accept that the authors themselves were about something other than giving us the true 'facts'. They are theologians, using the language of symbol and poetry to develop their great themes. Luke, when he tells the story of the coming of the Spirit, does so in language that links the experience to the God of the Hebrew Scriptures. Pentecost is the feast of the giving of the Law, and we are on Mount Sinai with Moses and Elijah, with the wind and the fire. We are encouraged to see the reversal of the Babel of Genesis in the gift of tongues, with the hope of a new understanding and harmony for humanity. The alternative version from 'Sources Close to Jesus' links the experience of the Spirit to the person of Jesus. His new life is breathed directly to his friends. The atmosphere is quiet and intimate. The author seems to be saying, in contradiction to Luke, that it is the God experienced in Jesus, rather than the God of Sinai, who comes in the Spirit. At the very least, the more popular version of the coming of the Spirit should be supplemented theologically and devotionally by the other and not treated as if it did not exist.

It is possible, even likely, there is a historical basis to both of the accounts of the coming of the Spirit, though the fact that in some respects they rule one another out means that we should not look for strict historical accuracy in either. It is possible, however, to imagine different recollections of what happened on both occasions with resulting disagreements among the disciples as to when precisely the Spirit was given. Thus the Spirit is a spirit of alternatives. The Spirit that comes from Jesus does not encourage a monolithic religion. Unity would not have been such a problem within Christendom if this had been recognized. The variety of Christian expression in practice and insight down the centuries, opening up into even greater variety today, should have been a matter for celebration rather than angst. I am fond of John Tavener's music, and it seems to me inspired by the Spirit. I was, however, dismayed to hear John say, at a teach-in at St. Alban's Cathedral at which I was present, that there had been no good music since the Reformation (except Bach, he reluctantly conceded). To deny the inspiration of the Spirit in the great classical heritage of western music, and in jazz and pop, seems to me analogous to the denial of the Spirit by one group of Christians of the other, and I suspect comes perilously close to what Jesus meant by the sin against the Spirit. (I have heard that, more recently, John has begun to be less devoted to the Orthodox Church than he once was. I wonder if this means that his view of western music will also broaden out?)

The two accounts of the reception of the Spirit not only stand as alternatives – they illuminate one another. This is especially true in the aspect of inclusiveness, which is very strong in Luke's account. Rocky chose as his text for the Pentecost sermon, the book of Joel. He invited his hearers to see the events of that time as the fulfilment of Joel's prophesy in which God promises, "I will pour out my Spirit upon **all flesh**." (NRSV) The crucial 'good news' word **ALL** echoes the message of God's agent at the birth of Jesus, "I am bringing you good news of joy for **all** the people." (1Luke 2:10) Both texts anticipate Paul's hope for the final outcome of the good news, "**...all** will be made alive in Christ." (1Corinthians 15:22) From beginning to end the faith established in Jesus is a universal faith. The inclusiveness of the spiritual awakening does away with sexism, ageism and class distinctions. The Spirit is poured out on old and young, men and women, and even on slaves. The term 'all flesh', as opposed to watered down versions that talk of 'all people,' includes the rest of the created order. 'On every living thing' is the original sense if it is to be in line with the book of Joel where 'the good news' is addressed to animals and vegetation.

'Fields, don't be afraid, but be joyful and be glad because of all God has done for you. Animals, don't be afraid- the pastures are green; the trees bear their fruit, and there are plenty of figs and grapes.'(Joel 2:21)

The Day of Pentecost is thus, or should be, the feast of the environment, a nature festival even.

What a great text you chose, Rocky. But what did you do with it? You brought forth a spectacular and emotionally charged response. You skillfully played on the guilt feelings of your assembled audience, charging them with the responsibility of killing God's Chosen One, even those who had been far from Jerusalem at the time. You had them eating out of the palm of your hand, begging for relief from the weight you had put on them. "Friends, what can we do about it?" Rocky was given a blank cheque. So he filled it in with a hefty sum. "Leave all your wrong-doing behind" – sounds easy until you try it – "Be dipped" – that means making your support of Jesus public to the official clergy and the Roman authorities, marking you down as an enemy of state and society- "Then you will receive the gift of God's Spirit."

The appeal was effective – not with everybody perhaps, but with large enough numbers to be very impressive and to get the Church off the ground. Very likely the 'apostles' would have needed to hire the 'Embassy Baths' (Siloam) for a week, for their exclusive use! Yes, the Spirit used Rocky's sermon to bring people to God through Jesus, despite the sermon's inadequacies. That is the miracle of preaching. That Rocky's interpretation fell far short of the text probably went unnoticed at the time. Nevertheless, Rocky's provisos set in motion a tragedy that would work itself out slowly and painfully for the next two thousand years. To Joel's "I will pour out my Spirit on all flesh," Rocky pronounced instead, "I will pour out my Spirit on those who are suitably contrite and join the club." Rocky put a limitation on the numbers and types who would be able to call themselves Christians or feel comfortable within the system. Worse, perhaps, he introduced a perception of the Spirit's scope and operation that was limited to narrow ecclesiastical tramlines.

What did Luke think of Rocky's sermon, as later it was reported to him and he wrote it down? No doubt, like us, his attention was focused on the immediate results of Rocky's preaching rather than the small print of the text itself. Rocky's script was to be used again and again, with variations, by the new community. It had something of the manifesto about it. However, Luke in his gospel records, in his own special way, this saying of Jesus.

"You're a rotten lot, but you look after your children and give them the right things. God is the very best of parents. So when you ask for God's Spirit, you'll receive her." (1Luke 11:13) (There is a different version Matthew 7:11)

So Luke knew very well, in fact emphasized, that the gift of the Spirit was not conditional either on moral attainment or on the performance of religious rites. The gift of the Spirit could be

25

obtained simply by asking God for it!

This rather critical view of Rocky's sermon and its relationship to the gift of the Spirit, as portrayed by Luke, has a bearing on the interpretation of the alternative account in 'Sources Close.' There Jesus follows the physical act of breathing the Spirit into his friends by telling them they now have the ability to assure people of forgiveness or otherwise, as they choose. A large chunk of the Church has interpreted this as meaning that the choice is a real one. It gives the clergy great power if they can refuse forgiveness to anyone who does not give them obedience. But if we bring to this account the inclusive message of the book of Joel and the text with which Rocky began his sermon, then to use the gift of forgiveness as a power mechanism is a misuse. The gift of the Spirit is for everybody and for every living thing. She brings with her the assurance of forgiveness, which means that what God has made, God loves, accepts and renews. The task of the friends of Jesus is to make that message clear and plain to all, not to play cat and mouse. The words of Jesus that accompany the gift of the Spirit mean simply that if Jesus' friends do not proclaim this message of forgiveness, it will not be proclaimed. It is a positive duty, not an option. The words come from the one who said, "If you do not forgive others their wrongs, the Loving God will not forgive you your wrongs." (Matthew 6:14) Jesus understood that forgiveness is a two-way experience. You need the forgiving attitude in order to receive forgiveness. Otherwise you will not understand the process or its cost. There is therefore a strong parallel between the way Christians, beginning doubtless with the first 'apostles', have applied the instruction of Jesus to forgive as giving them the option of withholding forgiveness, and the way Rocky put conditions on the reception of the Spirit at Pentecost.

If we are to be honest, then we must admit that not only in times past but still today the Church offers to the world a rather uncertain selection of goodies, which, moreover cannot be tasted or examined in detail until the money has been paid. The coinage

demanded is conformity. But very slowly, there is a new understanding of the Spirit emerging that is not happy with this market
practice. It certainly would not be accepted as best practice in the
commercial world where the customer is supposed to have
'rights'. Those who have difficulty in breaking free from sins of
an anti-social nature; those who have problems with items of the
creed or theological language; those who cannot sign on the
dotted line but see themselves as 'seekers' are still excluded from
the fortress of Christendom or regarded as second class citizens.
But some of us are beginning to realize it is time such people were
affirmed as sharing the divine nature, as having received the
Spirit poured on all at Pentecost, and as having, despite their
weaknesses (paralleled all too obviously by the weaknesses of
those who stand firmly on the rock) gifts, attributes and insights
to contribute to God's New World. Even this is only nibbling at
the text Rocky chose for his sermon. Those of other religions?
Those who produce, like Scorsese's film of Kazantzakis' novel
'The Last Temptation', works of art that challenge Christian
assumptions? The inarticulate and throttled cries of those pushed
to the margins of our society?

I was present at a huge ecumenical Pentecost service in
Westminster Cathedral in London in 1995. It marked an initiative
entitled "The Great Banquet" at which many groups and communities in the metropolis joined together to eat and drink.
Politicians sat next to drug addicts and so forth – well – just for
once. The service, at which there was a congregation of over
2,000, was rudely interrupted by a member of London's hungry
homeless up the front who shouted and screamed his anger at the
whole performance. The response of the church (probably
standard practice) was for the organist to play full blast (the
sound was truly deafening) while the offender was escorted out.
I am sure I was not the only one who was made to realize that
whereas we Christians thought we were doing something
tremendous – so ecumenical – a Baptist preacher and a

Pentecostalist gospel group in a Catholic cathedral, and the Salvation Army accompanying the singing with their band – to the hungry homeless we appeared smug and if not unsympathetic, then quite incompetent to do anything but tickle the problems they face, not just at Pentecost but day after day. He should have been handed the mike and we should all have had the opportunity to hear what he had to say, "Fs" and all. I suspect he would not have preached for as long as Eric Blakeborough, who later in the service preached to the point of the occasion and from his experience of getting alongside just such people. The interrupter may well have enjoyed Eric, especially the humorous bits, and may well have come to realize that there are Christians genuinely on his side. But he was excluded by the machine from speaking and then from listening. On the Day of Pentecost 1995, The Holy Catholic and Apostolic Church in one of its wider manifestations did a Rocky and failed to acknowledge the Spirit blowing from outside it fences.

He is Alive

(1) He is alive! Time to rejoice!
Now is the day to find your voice;
Tell every culture, every creed,
"The one you seek is risen indeed!"

(2) He is alive! Who then shall fear
To face life's challenges and care?
Or make their feelings truly known
To him who craves no crown or throne?

(3) He is alive! The verdict stands-
You are set free by nail-pierced hands;
Justice more kind than courts decide,-
A judge who takes the offender's side!

(4) He is alive! The barriers fall;
The Holy City welcomes all;
Villains and victims, straight and queer,
All now to one another dear.

(5) One world -a dream beyond all hope
Jesus has brought within our scope;
You know his love, you know his name,-
So sing along and spread his fame!

(After Josiah Conder 1789-1855'The Lord is King! Lift up thy voice.' Tunes: Niagara or Church Triumphant.)

Chapter Four

SIMON, SIMON.....!

A married couple, Nye and Sapphire, sold some of their property. Nye made out he was bringing all the money from the sale to the leaders, but actually kept some of it back. His wife knew what he was up to. Rocky challenged him, "Nye, why are you behaving in such an evil way? You've pocketed part of the money you got from the sale of your property!Do you think you can play a trick on God's Spirit? It was your property before you sold it, and afterwards you were free to do what you liked with the money. Why all this deceit? It's not us you're trying to cheat, but God!" Rocky's words caused Nye to have a heart attack, and he collapsed dead on the floor. Everybody who got to hear about it was very shocked. Some of the younger people took charge, wrapped him in a sheet, and took him away to be buried.

About three hours later, Sapphire arrived, not knowing what had happened. Rockychallenged her. 'Did you and your husband sell your land for the amount you told me?" "Yes" she said, "that's what we got from the sale." Rocky said, "Why did you two plan together to find out if God's Spirit could catch you cheating? The people who've just buried your husband will be back any minute for you!" She then collapsed in front of him and died. The young people came in, made sure she was dead, then carried her out to bury her beside her husband. The members of the church and others who got to hear about it were very frightened. 2Luke 5: 1-11.

I cannot really remember when my passion for history began. But it was greatly stimulated at the age of ten by visits to an old blind man, Mr. Kingdom, who lived in the flat above the draper's shop kept by his daughter Phyllis, opposite the War Memorial, in Ilfracombe where I spent part of my childhood. Mr. Kingdom used to get me to read to him popular schoolboy-type history and gave me my first history book *'Kings and Queens of England'*.He was particularly interested in the reign of Elizabeth and he taught me to admire her brilliance in matters of state and her inspiration to her people to perform feats of nobility and heroism. But when we came to the tragic story of Mary, Queen of Scots, he shook his head sadly and said, "That was the one great blot on her copybook."

If asked to identify the one great blot on Rocky's copybook, most people averagely familiar with the scriptures would cite without much hesitation his three-fold denial of Jesus. But for my money it would be his treatment of Nye and Sapphire. His denial was an act of human weakness. His treatment of the shifty couple was an act of religious heavy handedness. There can be no doubt which category Jesus regarded as the more serious. Nye and Sapphire were two recent converts to the faith from the middle classes, tarred with middle class attachment to material things and adequate insurance cover. They come across as shallow and inconsistent rather than wickedly dishonest, meriting a good talking to, but hardly deserving capital punishment!

To be fair to Rocky, he had some job on his hands. A Galilean fishmonger suddenly the head of a community of three thousand plus – keen, enthusiastic converts from all social classes – that fact in itself a threat to the established order. Some were used to being bowed and scraped to by the masses, others ignorant and uncouth, heads buzzing with all manner of notions, some ideal- istic, some idiotic. Some were convinced they were the sole possessors of absolute truth, others ready to experiment in a new-found freedom. Cheery, for example, felt inspired to place his considerable wealth 'at the apostles' feet'. Perhaps he knew the story of the 'rich young ruler', even knew him personally since they probably belonged to the same social set. Cheery took the words of Jesus about selling everything and giving to the poor as a command for himself. Whether this was what the apostles wanted we do not know. To be suddenly the trustees of vast capital resources was yet another weighty responsibility on their shoulders. The impression we get is that this movement was a voluntary one. No one was obliged to fall in behind Cheery. The wrong of which Nye and Sapphire were convicted was not the holding back of part of their capital, but telling lies about it. On the other hand we can imagine the immense moral pressure there must have been to cough up. It would probably have been difficult for someone known to have financial assets tucked away to be accepted as a Christian 'first-class'.

The whole operation must have been difficult to keep under control, practically and emotionally. There had to be some discipline! (Did there?) Luke's account makes it clear that the harsh disciplining of Nye and Sapphire was a warning to all those tempted to exploit the newness and uncertainties in the early Christian community by getting up to any kind of hanky-panky. Indeed, some would say that if Rocky had not made some such example as this, the Church might have fallen apart and not survived.

What did Rocky do to Sapphire and Nye? Quite literally, he frightened the life out of them! It sounds incredible that Rocky's stern words should cause husband and then later wife to have a heart attack. In the 1970s, a meek and mild Westminster M.P., Hugh Delargy, died of a heart attack while facing a vicious barracking from the opposing benches. His colleagues, in the heat of the event, accused their opponents of murder. In more primitive times this type of thing was not at all uncommon. The witch doctor in Africa can still do it – pick out guilty people from a circle and kill them with a look.

Simon, Simon…how could you? Just listen to him! "Nye, why are you behaving in such an evil way?…Do you think you can play a trick on God's Spirit?"Had Rocky never lied? Had Rocky never fallen victim to temptation's power?(See 1Luke 22:54) In the courtyard of Guy's Palace, Rocky was given the opportunity three times to resist the temptation to deny any relationship with Jesus. Nye and Sapphire were only given one chance each to tell the truth. Rocky lied with gusto, spicing his protestations with rich Galilean oaths and curses. Nye and Sapphire merely indulged in the right, as they saw it, to respond with misinformation when their private affairs were being invaded.

Simon, Simon...told by Jesus to forgive 'seventy times seven', and to these first offenders you mete out the maximum penalty! (Matthew 18:21 & 1Luke 17:3) Simon, Simon, who in the courtyard caught that look of Jesus, the look of love and forgiveness that drove you to tears- you gave to Nye and Sapphire the look that killed.

This regrettable, no, damnable incident should serve to teach us to look for leadership, example and inspiration to Jesus. There are perils in looking elsewhere, even to the apostles. Those who base their theology and morality on the teachings of Paul, great Christian commentator though he was, are in danger of kicking off with a second-hand Christianity. Paul, on his own admission, only possessed a partial knowledge.

'Everything we know is a tiny fraction of what there is to know; in our deepest understanding of events we only scratch the surface.'

'What we know now is like seeing a blurred reflection in a piece of shiny metal.' (From 1Corinth 13)

The writer of 'The Call to Trust' (Letter to the Hebrews) was possibly Cilla, a friend of Paul. She tells us,

'Let's keep our eyes on Jesus our coach. He knows the course from experience...Think of the example Jesus set you.' (Chapter 12)

Keep your eyes on Rocky and you will come to the conclusion

that it is alright to go around giving people heart attacks if you think they are wickedly frustrating God's purposes. Even if you hesitate to follow the example of Rocky to the letter in this respect, you may nevertheless be inspired to defend your faith in an aggressive, inhuman, love-less way.

The blot on Rocky's copybook also reminds us of how easily we judge others when we are guilty ourselves, often of the same offence. I remember hearing on a Sunday morning Christian program a new convert being interviewed. He had received a vision calling him to go through the streets of Soho (London's 'red light' district) with a banner denouncing 'Sin', by which he meant 'Sex'. One didn't have to be a psychiatrist to realize that he had a sex problem himself. But instead of this helping him to be sensitive and understanding in regard to the weaknesses of others, he sought to conceal his own state by pointing the finger elsewhere. He did not fool me, nor the experienced eyes in Soho, I warrant, though perhaps he fooled a few Christians into thinking him very brave! "Anyone who has never done anything wrong can throw the first stone!" Jesus said. Rocky had forgotten those words, spoken when a woman caught committing a sexual offence had been brought before Jesus for judgment. The prose-cutors on that occasion had slunk away one by one, the eldest first. The words of Jesus are a call to us to pause and consider whether it is not we ourselves who merit the penalty or rebuke we are so quick to give to another. ('Sources Close' 8: 1-11)

There is something yet more serious to consider. We have before us the story of the death of two people, a husband and wife. They were seen by Rocky as expendable. (Otherwise, after what happened to Nye, he would have been more careful with Sapphire!) The Church, thought Rocky, would be better off without them! Can we really imagine this to be so? Had Sapphire and Nye no good qualities? Had they nothing to offer? What had brought them to Jesus in the first place? Mixed motives if they were like the rest of us, which means good as well as bad, not just bad as well as good.

The story of the contest between Elijah and the prophets of Baal on Mount Carmel is a favorite story for many people. Remember the sequel? Having proved his point that the God of Israel could bring fire from heaven whereas Baal from Syria could not, the 450 prophets of Baal and the 400 prophets of Asherah were taken on Elijah's orders down the brook Kishon and killed. What a tragedy! 850 potential converts – a trained body of clergy who had seen the wonders of the true God and could have been banded into a missionary team to take the message to the ends of the earth – wiped out at a stroke! No wonder shortly afterwards Elijah is described as having a fit of depression and loss of nerve. Perhaps he realized what a blunder he had made. (1Kings 18: 1-40 & 19:5)

I am reminded also of Mrs. Bevan (not her real name) who lived on the housing estate where I ministered for seven years. Mrs. Bevan was a large woman. She had been in prison several times and people were afraid of her. Somehow she and I got on well. She always sent me a Christmas card. Whenever we met in the street we stopped for a chinwag and especially when we chatted in the shop folk looked aghast, for we engaged in a teasing banter. "I'd come to your church, just for you, lovely boy" she said on one occasion, "except that the lot you've got there are too respectable!""We shan't be very respectable if *you* come," I said, and she laughed! But it was no laughing matter really. For if Mrs. Bevan had turned up she wouldn't have had much of a welcome, and she knew it. And that was a tragedy. Because Mrs. Bevan had a beautiful singing voice. She toured the clubs, where she was not really appreciated by the clientele, who didn't really mind what the act was like after they had partaken of a few pints. But she had enough pride in her performance to take up lessons with an international opera star who lived locally. The singing in our little church was often abysmal and we had to disband our choir for want of talent. The singing would have improved one hundred per cent if Mrs. Bevan had joined us.

The Church brings poverty on itself by consigning people to the dustbin. No, Rocky, you did not do well, and we do not do well to follow you.

Luke tells the story of Nye and Sapphire po-faced. He plays the objective historian who gives us the facts without any particular turn of phrase to provide praise or blame. He keeps his comments for afterwards. These comments provide the vital clues to Luke's attitude. First Luke tells us that *fear* fell on the whole church. Was fear the emotion the Good News was intended to generate? It is Luke who records in his 'part one' the proposal by 'Thunder and Lightning' (Jim and John) to call down fire from heaven on a Samaritan village that had refused to give Jesus hospitality. Luke tells us,

But Jesus gave them a stern talking to. He said, "You must put a stop to those angry feelings of yours. The Complete Person doesn't set out to kill people, but to bring them to life." 1Luke 9:51

The clear implication of this story, and the clear motive for telling it, is that fear of punishment is not to be used as a method of evangelism. It is also Luke who records the story of the tearaway lad who was so afraid of the reception he would receive from his father on returning home that he planned to offer to do unpaid work on the farm. Had his fear been greater, it might have prevented his return. But his father embraced him before he had chance to make the offer. The good news of the father's love is portrayed by Jesus in order to banish the fear of those who suspect they might get less than gentle treatment if they decide to come home to God.

Luke has one more damning comment to make in respect of this incident. *'People who were not members of the group were too frightened to join them, though they talked of them with respect.'* The second part of this comment is perhaps even more telling than the first. People spoke well of the Christian community *despite* the action of Rocky, not because of it! There were Christians in the early Church who continued to impress outsiders by their life of love. But behavior like that of Rocky stood as a barrier to prevent that love from drawing other people into the fellowship. Anyone who believes that fear can be an element in effective evangelism should take careful note of what Luke is saying. The movement that began with the mass dipping at Pentecost and in which Rocky played such a leading part, was now brought to an end. Fear brought evangelism to a screeching halt. Only persecution and scattering and a new approach to people of other cultures and types would get things going again. It is Luke the Greek, the outsider, who groans, "Ticket holders only from now on!" This has great significance for our times. Luke informs us that while the infant institutional 'Church' made no new members because people were frightened by those in charge, yet *'Despite this, the numbers of those who put their trust in Jesus, the Leader, continued to grow, women and men.'*

In the last fifty years of the last century great swathes of the Christian churches were taken over by fundamentalism of varying kinds, Catholic, Protestant, Pentecostalist, and fringe Sectarian. Not all fundamentalists are nasty. Many have hearts much larger than their theology. But the overall impression given by churches and groups with the fundamentalist virus is that they are out to control and manipulate, terrorize and oppress the lives of people. They dictate the thoughts, the behavior, the life-style of those they get their grips on in an unpleasant way. It is the religion of fear. The word love is bandied about, but it is about as appropriate in some quarters as in 'The Ministry of Love' in George Orwell's 1984. Indeed, as far as the Christian Church is concerned, Orwell was not far out in his timing. Witness the disgraceful, un-Christlike, scripturally unenlightened attitude the Church presents to the world in respect of gay people. Though fuelled by the fascist right, this attitude spills right across the middle-ground and beyond, so that the churches are paralyzed and unable to make a loving, informed response. Most western societies increasingly understand gay sexuality, accept it and appreciate its valuable contribution to community and culture. Only the Church and mindless thugs maintain their ignorance and opposition. Intelligent, kind, caring people outside the Church are mystified and repelled by the Church's outdated and irrelevant debates. So while respect for Jesus and his message continue among the population as a whole, church membership continues to decline. When Jesus is turned out of his Church, then Jesus finds his friends outside.

And so, in very few words, but with sufficient clarity for those on the look out, Luke records the dramatic lurch from the mind and will of Jesus to the mind and will of the Church as it has happened many times throughout the centuries. "You can come in if you are one of us and if you behave and believe like us. If not, we have ways of keeping you out." "We will preach love, but if anyone gets too near to practicing it, we know where to draw the line!"

Should Luke have made his point more clearly and effectively? He surely thought he was being clear and plain enough for anyone who knew Jesus –either first hand or by drinking from his spirit. He would probably be disappointed, as many a preacher has been, at the way in which his hearers manage somehow to adopt the very line of conduct he was seeking to dissuade them from taking. The ability of Christians to listen, Sunday by Sunday, to good news and then translate it for the purpose of distribution to the world into bad news, is amazing. It is 'rock hard' Simon the Church has chosen to emulate, rather that the one who 'went about doing good.' The 'bad acts' continue.

*ONWARD CHRISTIAN COMRADES**

(1) Onward, Christian comrades*,
Jesus shows the way;
With his cross to guide us,
Love will bring the day.
Face with good each evil,
Wrath with the soft word,
Smile till stone-faced bigots
Meekly drop their guard.

Chorus: Onward, Christian...

(2) Feeling for each other,
Freely let us move,
Sisters, brothers, partners
In the cause of love;
Celebrating difference,
Recognizing worth;
No one is rejected,
No one trapped by self.

Chorus...

(3) Crowns and thrones must perish,
Power blocks all fall;
One foundation constant,
God's strong love for all;
Ignorance and prejudice
Try to undermine,
God still goes on loving
Past the end of time.

Chorus...

39

(4) Onward, freedom-seekers,
Set your souls at ease;
You will be composers
Of new harmonies:
Glory without triumph,
Prize with none's defeat;
First the first place taking,
Washing others' feet.

Chorus...

(After Sabine Baring-Gould 1834-1924. Tune: St. Gertrude –
Sullivan. Faint hearts worried about the word 'comrade' may
sing instead, "Onward, Christians, onward..."

Chapter Five

WHAT DO WE DO WITH THEM?

'At the same time as the followers of Jesus were growing in number, those whose first language was Greek complained they were being discriminated against by those who spoke the Jewish language. They thought their people who had no means of support from a family were not getting their fair share in the food handed out each day. The twelve leaders called everybody together and said, "We've got enough to do telling people the truth about God, without having to act like waiters. So friends, we suggest you chose seven responsible people to be in charge of this work. They must have the right motives and carry the respect of everybody. We will spend our time keeping in touch with God and passing on what God has to say." Everybody thought this made sense, so they chose Steven, known for his strong convictions and closeness to God, and with him Philip, Russ, Nicky, Tim, Craig and Colin (a convert to the Jewish religion from Antioch). These were introduced to the leaders, who asked God to help them and gave them a hug. God's message reached more and more people, and there were new followers joining all the time, including many of the temple clergy.' Luke's Good News Part Two (Acts) 6: 1-6.

I remember John Williams Hughes, one-time Principal of Bangor Baptist College, making a 'thank-you' speech to the ladies who had provided refreshments at a gathering of ministers in a chapel in Pontypridd sometime in the late 1960s. In Wales there is a tradition of very generous provisions on such occasions, indeed chapels vie with one another in 'putting on a spread'. The thank you speeches are no less a tradition – English immigrants find them tedious. Always two speakers are chosen to say thank you. There used to be some ministers who specialized in the art. The 'proposer' and 'seconder' of the thanks are expected to go over the top in their praise of the good works that have resulted in their replenishment, and they are also expected to be witty! The ladies are invited to come out of the kitchen to listen. Williams Hughes was something of a saint, a warm hearted man, an entertaining preacher with a quiet style of his own, a cunning critic from within of the less endearing aspects of Welsh chapel life, endowed with a wicked but not cruel sense of humor. I don't remember the anecdotes with which he entranced his audience on this occasion, only his final words. "GOD BLESS THE LADIES! WE CAN'T DO ANYTHING WITHOUT THEM, (pause) AND WE CAN'T DO ANYTHING WITH THEM!"

The ministers (all male) laughed. They understood the joke! The women smiled indulgently and one of their number graciously replied, as part of the tradition. Williams Hughes' remark was not meant to be unkind, indeed was not meant to be anything in particular other than a sharp way of bringing a speech to an end. At this distance in time, however, it seems to be far from funny. It did and still does say a lot about the position of women in the Christian Church. It speaks of the continuous problem for the leaders of the Church that women represent such an overwhelming majority of churchgoers in many parts of the world, particularly in Europe. I was invited to a conference about that time which had the title 'Winning men for Christ'. Those attending would be provided with techniques that would enable them to bring in hordes of men to the churches, thereby adjusting this embarrassing imbalance. I did not attend the conference. Embedded in my memory is a rebuke I once received from another Welsh Baptist saint, Howard Williams. I wrote to him at Bloomsbury Central Baptist Church in the first year of my ministry in a vast barn of a chapel at the entrance to the Rhondda Valley. I knew him to be sympathetic to the struggles of those of us who were trying to stem the 'decline' in the Valleys. I complained that my congregation consisted largely of people over the age of sixty, and that these were nearly all women. I received from Howard a tender and encouraging letter. But he ended by saying, "Don't forget that the women were the first at the Resurrection." Not long after, those elderly women allowed me to train them in the latest techniques of visitation evangelism and they went out in twos several nights a week for a period of five years until the whole neighborhood had been covered again and again, with the result that at the end of those five years our numerical membership was identical to what it had been at the start. Those acquainted with conditions in the valleys at that time will realize this was quite a feat. All around us other chapels were declining and closing fast.

The early church did not know what to do with its women. The ministry of Jesus opened the floodgates and in poured a section of humanity that had hitherto been regarded as theologically irrelevant. From day one the church was faced with the difficulty of having as its most active, most loyal, most devoted, most enthusiastic and hard working members, people regarded as being the wrong sex for leadership or anything else of importance except, oh yes, motherhood!

Not only was the early church lumbered with a disproportionate number of women, many of these were widows and something of a drain on resources. There is no mention of widowers, since men found it easy enough to obtain another wife. The market was flooded with poor dears anxious to 'overcome their reproach'. Without a man they were nothing! Once a woman had lost her youthful looks and was no longer capable of bearing children she was regarded by the society of the day as valueless. Even a church running away as fast as it could from the attitude of Jesus to women could not regard anyone as valueless. So widows were given a particular status. They could pray! Though not, of course, in the corporate gatherings of the church where men were present!(See the first of two imaginary letters from Paul to his friend Timothy 5:5 and Paul's first letter to the Christians of

Corinth 14: 34)

Against this background, with which he was all too familiar, Luke reports a bit of a fracas among the widows. Whether the complaint of the Greek-speaking Jewish Christians against the Jewish-speaking Jewish Christians that there was unfairness in the provision of food had any validity, Luke does not tell us. He is not interested in that point. What he does succeed in making clear is that the apostles were accused of not being fair – that is, not doing their job effectively – and that the women's section was up in arms. Something needed to be done.

A grand meeting of the Jerusalem Christians was called. We must presume that one of the apostles had been briefed by the others to speak on their behalf. He began with the astounding statement, which does not seem to have been challenged:

"We've got enough to do telling people about God, without having to act like waiters."

Looked at from one angle the statement represents an admission from the apostles that they were not coping. "We can't do anything with them!" From another angle it represents another retreat from the teaching of Jesus, so often and so painstakingly given them, on one occasion with a towel and basin. Luke may not have known about that acted parable, but he did know Jesus had said,

*"...anyone who thinks they have leadership qualities must show they are not above doing the dirty jobs. The needs of the customers in a restaurant come before the needs of the waiter. I'm showing you how to act like the perfect waiter."*1Luke 22: 26.

Religious functions, which the apostles produce as an excuse for ducking their responsibilities, were, in the mind of Jesus, inseparable from humble obedience. Like the priest and the Levite in the story of the 'Good Samaritan', the apostles do not think they should allow themselves to be distracted from their prime calling to attend to those in difficulty by the wayside. Someone of a lesser breed can see to that sort of thing.

Thus it takes only six chapters into Luke's second volume to identify that point at which begins the separation between clergy and laity that most Christians still take for granted. In the arrangements that follow, without any debate about the principle of the thing, we see the commencement of the process of creating a terraced structure within the Church. Two distinct tiers of ministry emerge, to be followed in the course of history by further gradations. Some Christians still think these distinctions to have been ordained by Jesus himself. It is doubtful whether Luke thought so. Significantly, he makes no mention of the Spirit as the inspiration for the new arrangements as he does when a later meeting of leaders makes provision for Gentiles to join the Church. (2Luke 15:28) If Jesus intended a separate ministry at all, then he intended it as a ministry of service in which presenting the Good News and the alleviating of physical distress go hand in hand. (1Luke 9). We can be quite certain Jesus did not advocate a career structure. Yet that is what we have in most churches today – there is no mistaking it. The secular world recognizes its own patterns of promotion and status in the structure of the Church. According to Luke, the apostles are to blame for this deviation from the mind of Jesus.

It is interesting to speculate what would have been the pattern of church life subsequently if, instead of creating a class of lower-ranking officers to do the chores, the apostles had established a rota system whereby all church members took it in turn to 'act as waiters'.

But we must return to the problem that brought the call for radical re-organization- the women! The women were getting out of hand; they were making complaints. Under the guidance of the apostles, the Christian community chose seven **men** to supervise the women's work and other such irksome tasks, while the apostles held the limelight. The women were not considered capable enough to manage their own affairs. Since it was, we assume, the 'twelve' male apostles who had been failing to make a go of the charitable distribution among the women, why not let the women have a go?

In the first volume of Luke's work we find the pattern for what he would have regarded as a preferable outcome. In 6: 12 Luke gives an account of the calling by Jesus of the male apostles. But Luke, unlike the other gospel writers, in chapter 8 parallels this with the calling of the female apostles. These, like the men, are described as being 'on his team', (Greek: 'with him', one of the special marks of apostleship, see Mark 3:14.) Three (a holy number, like seven and twelve) are specifically mentioned by Luke, though he makes it clear there were more. The three mentioned, Maggie, Joan and Susan, were women of substance, able to support the group financially. They were probably more proficient in the matter of economics than the men, for at least one had experience of the management of Herod's court. Judas kept the purse, but in all probability Joan kept an eye on the books! These women coped well during the ministry of Jesus, and did not, like the men, do a bunk when things got tough. Some of them must still have been around when the men called the big meeting. They were Jesus' own chosen. Why were they not put in charge of the charity work? Indeed, why were they not already in charge?

In his unfolding of the story of the early Christian community, Luke makes it clear that the seven male 'helpers' chosen by the meeting could not be tied down to menial tasks. Steven and Philip were good at preaching and evangelism. Luke follows the call of the women apostles by the story of Mary and Martha (1Luke 10:38) where Martha is called to set on one side the household chores and become a theological student with her sister, 'at Jesus' feet'. Luke intends us to understand the story as the call of both Mary Dategrove and her sister Martha to the ranks of the apostles.

According to Luke, service and leadership are inseparable and in both women are meant to take their place with the men.

There is much in Luke's great two-volume work to indicate that Luke was a champion of the cause of women and that in this respect he knew he was following in the footsteps of Jesus. In Luke's day it proved to be a lost cause. But he made his protest, and we can pick up his banner and carry it forward.

DEAR SPIRIT OF GOD

Dear Spirit of God, our hearts inspire,
And warm and light them with your fire;
Of you we drink; our fervor lifts;
You shower us with such precious gifts.

When sick, with healing balm you soothe;
You make our weary muscles move;
And as we grope to find our way
You shine a torch as bright as day.

Blow fierce strong wind, knock barriers down;
Relax the good with singer and clown;
Then gentle, female dove proclaim
That peace which seasoned lovers claim.

Escort us to the home of God;
There show us how you play your part;
You Son and Father interface
And complement with mother's grace.

(Doxology) Praise life and love and power and voice,
Beauty and feeling, thought and choice.

(Button Polished. Veni Creator Spiritus)

Chapter Six

"OURS BE THE GLORY" and "YOU'D BETTER DO IT OUR WAY!"

Those who had been forced to leave their homes, spread their ideas wherever they went. Philip went to a town in Samaria and spoke to the people there about God's Chosen. Large crowds gathered and listened attentively to what Philip had to say. They were impressed by the remarkable things he was doing. People who had been mentally disturbed found peace, and some of the disabled, the arthritic, and the paralysed, were healed. The whole community shared in the happiness.

In the same town there was a famous magician, a popular entertainer, called Simon. Everybody took notice of him, including the leaders of the community. They believed his powers were supernatural. Simon's abilities as a magician were amazing. He had the power to hold people's attention for a long time. But their attention was now drawn to Philip and his good news about Jesus and God's New World. When women and men accepted what Philip had to say, they were dipped. Simon was one of these, and when he had been dipped he went everywhere with Philip. He was amazed by all the wonderful things he saw happening.

When the leaders back in Jerusalem heard the people of Samaria had accepted God's message, they sent Rocky and John to Samaria to find out the facts. The first thing they did when they arrived was to ask God to give the new converts the Spirit. Up to now God's Spirit had not entered any of them. Only the name of Jesus the Leader had been used when they were dipped. Rocky and John hugged each of them and they received God's Spirit.

When Simon saw people could get the Spirit just by being touched by the leaders, he said to them, "I'd like to be able to pass on God's Spirit by touching and hugging people. How much do you want?" But Rocky said, "Get out of my sight! And you can take your money with you! God's gifts aren't for sale! You're not one of us. You haven't got the right attitude. You'd better change from your bad ways and beg God to forgive your unworthy thoughts, if you can. I can see you're a thoroughly bad lot" Simon said, "Please speak to Jesus for me, so I escape the dangers you talk about." 2Luke (Acts) 8: 4-25.

The 'apostles' inaugurated a career structure for the Church by ordaining seven men to attend to the more humble tasks. At least it should be noted in the apostles' favour that they regarded humble appointments as worthy of special acts of ordination. If we must have ordination, then everybody in the Church should be ordained and everybody's gift recognized in celebration.

However, the Spirit is not so organized. Luke shows his feelings about the matter by recording without delay the work of two of these humble servants, Steven and Philip. Both spectacularly failed to confine themselves to menial tasks. Steven was an attractive young man whose gifts as a speaker were quickly appreciated. The high profile he adopted led to conflict with his own Greek speaking Jewish community, and then with the Jewish clergy who had him arrested. Steven's defense marks him out as the first Christian theologian. He provided for the first Christians, at this point still all faithful Jews, the theological basis on which they could withdraw from Temple worship and break free from the idea that to be God's people was the same as belonging to the nation. Steven is honored by the Church for being the first Christian martyr. But Steven was not martyred for being a Christian but for being a radical, unconventional, troublesome Christian. Only in very exceptional circumstances do conventional Christians get martyred. It is our Bonhoeffers, Luther-Kings and Romeros who are the more likely martyrs. Steven demonstrated his faithfulness to the example of Jesus by praying a prayer of forgiveness for those who were doing the wrong, in marked contrast to the way Rocky ignored the principle of forgiveness in dealing with Nye and Sapphire. Yet Rocky and the other apostles had the audacity and arrogance to think that by their touch they could pass on some crumbs of their authority to Steven, to be used sparingly in ways they approved. We are not told where the apostles were or what they were doing when Steven was killed, but if they had been standing by, making a non-violent protest, Luke would have told us. They are conspicuous by their absence. The apostles no doubt had a sneaking admiration for Steven, but in their eyes he had gone beyond his brief. They did not even attend his funeral. It was left to an anonymous group of devout people to make the arrangements and to act as mourners.

The other 'helper' who stepped out of line was Philip. This was 'Philip the Evangelist', so called to distinguish him from 'Philip the Apostle' of whom we hear nothing in Luke's second volume. Steven provided the theological reasoning to enable Christian Judaism to break its dykes. It was Philip who boldly put the theology into practice. He took advantage of the scattering following Steven's death to launch out on a mission to the people of Samaria. There is no mention of any special authorization by the apostles. Philip just got on with it! His successful mission to these semi-heathen half-breeds, as strict Jews thought of them, was followed by his conversion of the Ethiopian courtier. (2Luke 8: 26-40) The Ethiopian was black and sexually deviant. Color prejudice seems to be more of a modern perversity. It was because the African was a castrated man that he was marked out as a Gentile destined to remain as such, for 'eunuchs' were excluded from Jewish worship. (Deuteronomy 23:1) One of the anonymous prophets of Babylon seems likely to have been a eunuch. Castration was the fate of the leaders of the Jewish community when exiled to Babylon. He foresaw a time when eunuchs and 'foreigners' and other categories of outcast would be included among God's people. (Isaiah 56:1-8) This was a vision for a future time. It helped Philip to take the radical decision to dip the black deviant since they read together from the very scroll that contained the prophet's promise. But what is most noteworthy is that Luke shows us it was Philip the helper, and not the apostles, who responded first to the call of Jesus to evangelize the peoples of other nations. (2Luke 1:8)

Furthermore, Philip required no special vision like the one Rocky had on the rooftop at Jaffa in order to overcome an inbred prejudice. (2Luke 10 & 11) Philip followed up his conversion of people in Samaria and the Ethiopian by a visit to Azotus, a centre of Philistine culture, and from there he passed on the Good News in all the coastal towns, which were mainly Gentile, as far as Roman Caesarea. 'Caesartown' was where the Centurion Cornelius (Neil) was stationed, and it seems more than likely that his appetite for the Good News was whetted by Philip. Rocky had simply to build on a foundation that had already been laid. Thus we see a pattern in the careers of both Steven and Philip. The apostles were dragged along, not quite screaming and kicking perhaps, into a more adventurous and embracing expression of Christianity by the people they regarded as in some sense their inferiors, at least in office and status.

Luke gives us a good picture of the tension, if not rivalry, between the apostles and their 'helpers' in the story of the conversion of Simon the Magician. Philip's mission to Samaria was going well. People eagerly accepted the message, and there were examples of healing of body and mind. Particularly impressed was Simon, a local wonder-worker who practiced on the borders of magic and quack religion. He probably possessed some psychic abilities which he complemented with a bag of tricks, and neither he nor his audience were quite sure whether he was providing entertainment or service of a spiritual nature – like the fortune-teller at the seaside, or some of our more colorful 'charismatic' evangelists! Was he Messiah? Or just Marvo?

Simon recognized he was outclassed by Philip in terms of wonder-working. But it is unfair to Simon to accuse him of 'if you can't beat-em, join-em', and a misreading of the text. Luke tells us that Simon accepted what Philip had to say and obediently responded to the invitation to be dipped. He was also very attached to Philip and after his act of public witness, Simon followed Philip around everywhere. We get the impression that Philip was not only an effective communicator, but also a good counsellor, sensitive and patient. There is no suggestion that he found the attentions of Simon irksome. More likely he regarded him as good leadership potential and willingly shared with him what he knew.

All was well until the apostles decided to interfere. Something was going on down in Samaria – better check that everything was being done decently and in order! So Rocky and John arrived to inspect. Inspectors always have to justify their existence. Rocky and John noted a serious deficiency in Philip's work. Well, it was only to be expected. Philip was only a 'helper', after all was said and done. His converts were not receiving the Spirit! Had Philip forgotten to lay his hands on them after they came up out of the water? Or didn't he regard it as important? Or he didn't like to, in case he was usurping the apostles' authority? Read the manual next time, Philip!

It cannot have been easy for the friends who had accompanied Jesus through the hard and often frustrating period of his ministry, and been through the trauma of his death and the shock of their own inadequacy. They had survived to set in motion a revolution and had shown courage in the face of bullying author-ities. They were now struggling to hold the movement together in such a way as would preserve the heritage of their Jewish faith and permit the new freedoms of the Good News. It cannot have been easy for them to be upstaged by newcomers more talented, more attractive and more enterprising than themselves. *They* were the apostles. They were the ones who were sent. Others were welcome to assist, to add encouragement and enthusiasm, but not to steal the show! The vicar who finds her popularity waning in favour of a young curate is in need of grace, especially if some suggest the youngster's spiritual qualities are in some way superior. "Saul has slain his thousands, and David his tens of thousands" – mischievous words. (1Sam 18:7) With the chaos caused by the flight of many Christians from Jerusalem after the death of Steven, and people like Philip taking the initiative, the apostles must have felt things slipping from their grasp. What do you do in that kind of situation? Rocky and John took control of the mission in Samaria, out of the hands of Philip, by implication casting doubts on the effectiveness of his work. Immediately Philip was moved from that region to the desert. We hear of him doing no more in Samaria, though the apostles do some preaching there on the way back to Jerusalem. However, it is not the apostles who tell Philip where to go, but a special messenger from God. Philip still has his hot line that bypasses the apostles and directs him straight to the Ethiopian. Philip's mission, despite healings and other remarkable events, had not been 'spiritual' enough for Rocky and John. They were looking to see the same pattern as the Day of Pentecost. New followers of Jesus were meant to receive the Spirit. They were meant to speak in a special holy gobble-de-gook or behave in an excited manner that would attract everybody's attention.

The apostles assumed that because the established pattern was not present, the experience of conversion followed by dipping was invalid or incomplete. It was to be some time before Paul suggested the Spirit could be identified, perhaps more surely, in other ways, - by 'love', 'joy' and 'peace'. (1st letter to Corinth chaps 12-14 & Letter to Celtic Christians/Galatians 5:22) Meanwhile, the apostles introduced a feature of Christian initiation that has persisted throughout the centuries. "You won't be a real Christian unless you do it our way!" I remember my feelings of superiority in my teens, when, on occasion, we Baptists would have joint meetings with the Methodists. Of course they were very nice people, even if they did go on a bit about John Wesley. They were trying so hard to be Christians. It was such a pity that none of them had been baptized the Jesus way!"

An intriguing question arises as to what Philip thought of the ecclesiastical fussiness of Rocky and John, because when he dips the African there is no mention of receiving the Spirit by the formal 'laying on of hands', and there is no Rocky or John or any other member of the original gang to do it. Philip did not suggest a return to Jerusalem to find an apostle. The man went back to Ethiopia, well out of the way of further apostolic interference. Luke's acquaintance with Paul's teaching is reflected in his remark that the new Christian continued on his way *full of joy*. Joy was one of Paul's 'fruits of the Spirit'. As far as Luke was concerned, and as far as Philip was concerned, the Ethiopian had the Spirit. But would this have been enough for Rocky and John? The answer is *no*. There had been joy in Samaria at Philip's preaching. But according to the apostles, no Spirit! We must also assume from Rocky's later struggles that he would have had problems in accepting the Ethiopian at this stage, especially in view of his sexuality. Thoughts of Jesus may have persuaded Rocky to step over the line even so. But all our instincts seem to tell us that Rocky had not yet sorted himself out sufficiently to be able to perform Philip's 'at the edge' type of ministry. We still have more little Rockys than Philips on our staff!

Bad acts that have implications for church history are bad enough. Bad acts that display an on-the-spot lack of Christ-likeness in dealing with an individual are worse. Simon the Magician was Philip's convert. Philip understood him and he was 'coming along nicely' with Philip as his friend. Rocky, however, dealt with him with the sensitivity of a sledgehammer. Whether he had time to learn of Simon's background or acquaint himself with Simon's particular difficulties of adjustment we cannot tell – it doesn't look like it. Simon has given his name to 'Simony', the sin of trying to buy a place in the Church with money. This is not fair. Simon did not want to become a bishop. He wanted to be able to pass on the joy he had experienced. He had, after all, made a career of entertaining people and bringing a little variety and color into their lives. To be able to pass on the gift of the Spirit would be to do this in a grander and nobler way. Rocky misunderstood, misapplying the teaching of Jesus that you cannot serve God and money. Rocky, who had started life with the name Simon, accused his namesake of having the wrong attitude, bad ways and unworthy thoughts.

Reading this story from Rocky's point of view rather than Luke's, later generations attributed to Simon the emergence of the Gnostic heresy. There is no historical basis for this legend. But if Simon did go off and found another, perhaps more loving, version of Christianity, no one ought to be surprised. Luke's account gives no indication of anything of the kind happening. Luke's view is clear throughout the narrative. Simon the Magician is a believer, he receives the Spirit with the other believers, and finally he humbly asks Rocky and John to pray for him. They should have asked Simon to pray for *them*, - a prayer for sensitivity, a prayer for strength to overcome the urge to interfere with somebody else's success.

MY GRACIOUS FRIEND

My gracious Friend, you merit well
Each loving action I can show;
I own it as my greatest thrill
Your roles to play, your mind to know.

What is my being but for you,
It's sure support, its noblest end;
Your ever loving face in view,
Helping the cause of such a Friend.

I would not seek self-centred joy,
Or thrive against another's good;
Nor future days or powers employ
Spreading a famous name abroad.

It's for my Leader I would live,
The one who for my freedom died;
Nor could a world united give
More happiness than at his side.

His work my wrinkled age shall bless
When youthful vigor is no more.
And my last hour in life confess,
His love has animating power.

(After Philip Doddridge 1702-51 'My gracious Lord, I own thy right...')

Chapter Seven.

'BLINDNESS TO THE SIGHTED'

*God's Spirit directed Cheery and Saul to the nearest port, where they caught the boat to Cyprus. They landed at Salamis and talked about God in the Jewish places of worship. John Mark went along to help.They went right across the island as far as Paphos. There they met a magician, a Jewish confidence-trickster known as *"Slippery Al". He hung around the governor of the island, George Paul. George Paul was an intelligent man, and he invited Cheery and Saul to talk to him about God. But Slippery kept interrupting and trying to put the governor off. Saul, who from now on called himself Paul, was inspired to look Slippery straight in the eye and say, "You little devil, you stand in the way of everything that's good. You're up to all sorts of tricks. When are you going to stop twisting God's truth into something crooked? I'm telling you, God's not going to let you get away with it! Let's see how you like being blind! No sunshine for you for a while!" Straightaway Slippery Al found himself in a thick fog, and everything went black. He had to grope about, trying to find somebody to hold his hand. The governor was impressed and put his trust in Jesus. Then Paul and his friends caught the boat back to the mainland and landed at Perga. But John Mark left them and went home to Jerusalem. 2Luke 13: 6-13. (Slippery Al = Elymas = 'Crafty'; George Paul = Sergius Paulus.)*

After a while, Paul said to Cheery. 'How about going back to all the towns where we spoke God's message, to see how the new Christians are getting on?" Cheery wanted to take John Mark with them, but Paul was against this, because Mark opted out of the previous venture part way. There were such bitter words between Paul and Cheery that they ended their partnership. Cheery teamed up with Mark and they took the boat to Cyprus. Paul asked Silas to be his companion. They set out together, and the Christians asked God to look after them. They started by visiting the churches in Syria and the districts beyond. 2Luke 15: 35-41.

For longer than I wished I kept up the habit of attending meetings of the more informal kind for the clergy, in those days known in sexist language as 'fraternals'. I did this despite (or because of?) the fact that the colleagues I met there found the views I expressed surprising. However, I am grateful for the toleration shown to me over many years, with a few best forgotten exceptions, and I often benefited not only from the company – sometimes we became almost human – but also for the comeback! At one of my very earliest such meetings the ministers were invited to share any 'embarrassing moments' they had experienced in the course of their duties. I have returned many times to one of the shared experiences, hoping to keep its lesson close to heart. The minister had been visiting a church as a guest preacher for the first time. He took with him a sermon of which he was very proud, having re-worked, embellished and polished it often. It was a sermon on the healing of the blind man by Jesus. After the service he was told that there had been a blind man in his congregation. Our friend described how in one moment his pride and confidence in the excellence of his sermon collapsed, and how he felt a complete worm. I relive the experience with him to remind myself of how easy it is to set forth truths, sound enough in themselves, in a manner that demonstrates you have never entered into the real live situations they relate to, nor exercised your imagination to that end. John's Gospel (Sources Close) kickstarts the process of relating the story of the blind man to moral and spiritual blindness for which Jesus is healing and light. Jesus himself referred to the strict set as 'blind guides' *"Get knotted, you blinkered know-alls!"* (Good News from a Jewish Friend [Matt]:23: 16.) He pronounced them guilty of being over-confident of their clear-sightedness. (Sources Close 9:41) Someone who is physically without sight is justified in protesting, 'Don't forget me!' Proclaim that a simple act of 'trusting Jesus' will put every-thing right in the presence of a drug addict, a compulsive gambler or a habitual sex offender or to someone committed to befriending such people and you will distress or annoy, though you deserve a more violent reaction. I like to think that Dr. Luke shared to some degree the frustration and unhappiness of his patients when their ailments were resistant to his medicines, and that in recording the medical successes of Jesus he entered imagi-natively into the joy of patient and doctor.

One of Dr. Luke's patients was Paul. It was Paul who called him 'Beloved Physician'. We do not know for sure what Paul's ailments were or whether one of them was the stubborn 'thorn in the flesh' which resisted cure, or whether it was a 'side of his personality he was not at ease with' (GAN pg 356) We know he had trouble with his eyes, on at least one occasion experiencing temporary loss of sight. His need for a team of secretaries and the large print with which he signed his name (GAN pg 385) suggests a continuing problem. It was Paul's spiritual pilgrimage that led him to believe there was a connection between his physical and spiritual ills. The 'thorn in the flesh' was a discipline to prevent him from getting too big for his boots. His loss of sight on the Damascus Road was inseparable in his own mind from the blind fury with which he had pursued the Jesus people of Jerusalem to prison and even death. The scales that fell from his eyes at the healing touch of Ian (Ananias) correspond with his conversion. Only someone who has lost their sight can enter into the fear, the isolation, the bitterness of Paul's experience. Only someone who has temporarily lost their sight can enter into the elation of the moment when Paul found he could see again. However, there must always be a warning when there seems to be close corre-spondence between one person's experience and another's. "I know how you feel, I have been through it myself" can sometimes be a word of comfort. It is probably not the truth. No-one knows how you feel except you. You may go through similar experiences as another, but your feelings may be quite different. In any case we do not remember precisely what our feelings were at any one time – we have a remarkable forgettery in that respect. Certain things stand out and remain with us, but they may not be the things that were most urgent at the time – these we may have forgotten. In order to sympathize we must first recognize another person's separate identity and then listen very hard. Even then we may not hear or may not understand the language.

When Paul was confronted by the opposition of Slippery Al on the island of Cyprus, all the bells started ringing. Here was someone whose case was very like Paul's own prior to his conversion. Slippery was a Jew, a wonder-worker, intelligent and educated (for he impressed the governor, George Paul who, we are told, was an intelligent man.) But Slippery was stubbornly resistant to the truth, as Paul had been. Paul understood, or thought he did. If he had been through an experience of physical loss of sight that led to an awareness of his spiritual blindness, would this not then be an appropriate road for Slippery to travel? *"Let's see how you like being blind! No sunshine for you for a while!"* Temporary loss of sight only, the exact experience Paul had been through. The reference to the sun is interesting, for it may have been the sharp rays of the sun that brought on Paul's blindness. Slippery was duly deprived of his sight and, like Paul on the Damascus Road, had to be led by the hand. We are not told whether Slippery continued sightless or whether anyone like Ian of Damascus was sent to instruct him. If he became a Christian we would probably have been told. If he did not then the comparison between Paul and Slippery breaks down and Paul is seen to have boobed badly. (The comparison breaks down earlier, for the bad language Paul used to Slippery, *"You little devil....etc*, is far removed from the gentle and pleading words of Jesus to Paul, *"Saul, Saul, why are you giving me all this hate?")* The Governor was impressed and became a Christian, though Jesus had something to say about those who depend on magic tricks for belief. (See

GAN pg.89)

What is Luke's opinion? As a Greek doctor his principles of healing were based on the principles of Hippocrates. The task of the doctor is to cure illness, not to inflict it. His own teaching he would have found confirmed by the practice of Jesus. We simply have to ask whether Luke could have imagined Jesus ever causing someone to lose their sight, even as a preliminary to conversion and faith. Luke alone of the gospel writers records the manifesto of Jesus proclaimed at Nazareth, the words of the prophet of Babylon,

> *God's Spirit has inspired me*
> *To bring the poor good news;*
> *She tells me, 'Get the blind to see,*
> *Bust the jails and set folk free;*
> *God's arms are open lovingly'.*
> (GAN pg. 189)

Luke also records Jesus giving sight to the man in Jericho, known to Mark as Barty Timson. Luke adds to Mark's description an account of the rejoicing of both the healed man and the people.

Paul's behavior, though it can be explained by his desire to put Slippery through the paces he himself had been through, with the resulting benefit, is none the less abominable. "Because the way was tough for me, I'm going to make it tough for you!" Many communities practice initiation ceremonies on those seeking to be accepted as full members. In tribal societies young adolescents may be put through tests involving physical pain and mental agony. Ceremonies based on the same principle survive in some institutions and in my father's day were common in theological colleges. It seems they still persist here and there in the armed forces. The argument for the retention of such practices is always the same. "I had to put up with it and it didn't do me any harm." Who says? The way to faith and to full health of body, mind and spirit is often a painful one. But it is not the calling of the Christian to supply the pain. It is our calling to relieve pain wherever possible and to bring it to an end. The fact that we have suffered the same or worse in our time should motivate us to that end. The infliction of guilt with its manifold side-effects on the would-be pilgrim, is a game the Church has played for too long and been allowed to get away with. "Just because I have never had the climate in which I could be honest about my sexuality, just because I have been made to feel ashamed of my thoughts and desires, just because I have kept it all under wraps so that I am often difficult and unpleasant, I am going to make sure *you* don't have any easy ride!" "We were never allowed to be ourselves; why should you be?"Jesus came to give sight to the sightless and to set the captive free, not to exchange one set of chains for another, nor to provide a false cloak of holy conviviality to hide deep wounds and a sense of shame.

Luke does not directly voice his disapproval of Paul's treatment of Slippery. But it may be that indirectly he records the disapproval of someone else.

Paul was the leader of the missionary team to Cyprus. The team included Cheery (Barnabas) and Cheery's nephew or cousin, John Mark. John Mark was more likely than not the author of the first gospel. His parents' house seems to have been the center of the Jerusalem Jesus people, containing the upstairs function room, scene of the 'Last Supper'. Mark was also probably the 'young man' who lost his clothing in the garden when Jesus was arrested, which means he would have had recollections of Jesus visiting his home. A young boy he may have been, but the young are impressionable and he can hardly have failed to have caught something of the excitement of the movement of which Jesus was the center. In particular he would have been hyper-aware of the events of the death and reported return to life of Jesus, as was the whole population of Jerusalem. Either at the feet of Jesus himself or at the feet of his parents, he would have become aware of the basis principles on which the ministry and mission of Jesus were founded. He had the edge on Paul when it came to first-hand knowledge of Jesus. The theologian tutored by Liam (Gamaliel) would be unlikely, however, to seek enlightenment from an immature youngster. Immediately after the incident with Slippery Al and the conversion of the Governor, Paul and his missionary team sailed from Cyprus to continue their mission on the mainland of Asia Minor (modern Turkey).

It is at this point that Luke records that John Mark dropped out and made his way home. When next Paul put a missionary team together he flatly refused to include Mark and this led to a sharp disagreement with Cheery, which ended by Paul taking a new companion, Silas, who went with him back to Asia Minor, while Cheery and Mark returned to Cyprus. What was this quarrel all about? Was Mark a deserter? Did he get cold feet? Was he prone to home-sickness? That's the most popular explanation. It makes a good story. Mark, the coward, who eventually is found back with Paul again, facing the perils of Rome, and hastily putting the finishing touches to his gospel prior to martyrdom, perhaps not even managing to finish chapter sixteen before the soldiers come and take him away! Another theory suggests a theological difference on the lines of Gentile versus Jew or freedom versus the Law – the usual point of difference between Paul and other Christians. Was Mark a strict Jew who objected to the conversion of a Roman consul? Luke records Mark's departure from the team as immediately following on the conversion of George Paul. Luke seems to be telling us something that to him was more obvious than it is to us. All explanations are speculative. But no more speculative than any other explanation is the possibility that Mark left the team because he was unhappy at the treatment of Slippery Al. Mark found that he could not reconcile Paul's actions with his memories of Jesus. If Paul was going to continue the practice of inflicting physical punishments on those who failed to respond to the message, as a technique of evangelism, then Mark wished to be counted out. Paul, like many great leaders, found criticism hard to take. However, it may be that Mark's protest was not entirely in vain since Luke provides us with no further examples of similar practice on the part of Paul. At the same time, Paul was unable to forgive Mark for drawing attention to his lack of likeness to Jesus. It is indeed often much easier to forgive someone for being wrong than for being right.

There are some interesting sequels to this story. First, it is highly significant that Cheery and Mark head back for Cyprus. If Mark was convinced that a wrong had been done, then he was the best person to put it right. Perhaps he thought to do for Slippery Al what Neil had done for Paul and minister to him the healing of body and spirit promised by implication when Paul said the loss of sight would be temporary. If so, Mark may have been disappointed. Alas, most of the messes Christians make are not put right so easily. It is also significant that Paul chose not to go back to Cyprus, if deep down he accepted Mark's view that he had dishonored Jesus there. Pilgrims, in being aware of imperfections are often best advised to put the past behind and set their sights on the future. (Letter to Philiptown chapter 3 GAN pg. 391)

The other sequel lies further in the future. Paul was reconciled to Mark- how and where we do not know. But in one of the scraps from Paul's letters that are worked into the non-authentic 'Second letter to Timothy', Paul asks specifically for Mark to be brought to him 'because he is such a valuable assistant.' Then we find Mark either in prison with Paul or allowed to attend to his needs there, and in the team letter to Quaketown and in the more personal letter to Phil, Ava and Captain Rider, Mark and Luke join Paul in sending greetings. The fact that Luke and Mark knew one another very well should set the imagination racing. Those who pore over the Greek, wrestling with the 'synoptic problem', fail to take this sufficiently into account. It may be that Luke had no need to 'make use of' Markan material in a manner suggestive of plagiarism. Mark may have loaned Luke his notes! By this time

Luke would also have some jottings of his own for his first draft of an account of the life of Jesus and might easily have asked Mark for permission to include in his own work what Mark had achieved so far. We ought not to think of Luke and Mark on the lines of contemporary writers of hymns, more concerned about copyright and protecting their profits than the spread of the truth the hymns contain. Mark probably inspired Luke, and inspired him moreover to think he could do even better. But they were not competitors, rather working for the same firm.

Did Luke and Mark discuss what happened on the island of Cyprus? They must have done. Perhaps when Paul was out of earshot. "How shall I tell that story, Mark?" "Tell it just as it was, Luke. With the help of God's Spirit, future friends of Jesus will know what to make of it." Some day, Mark, some day!

The God of Jesus

(1) The God of Jesus praise,
The God whose name is Love,
The One who speaks to every race,
All worth above.
'I am just what I am',
To Moses God confessed;
See Jesus, God in human frame,
To know the rest.

(2) The God of Jesus praise,
The God with friends galore,-
Boaz and Ruth in ancient days,
And many more.
The 'Shield' of Abraham,
Great David's 'Shepherd-King',
Ezekiel's 'Storm', Isaiah's 'Lamb',
Your praise we sing.

(3) It must be understood,
This God embraces more-
Inspiring Islam's brotherhood
And Buddha's lore.
Great thinkers seek the tracks
Of genius divine,-
The God of Darwin and of Marx,
Freud and Einstein.

(4) God summons us to song,
To vocalize our praise,
Enthuse with fiddle, drum or gong,
And lilting phrase.
Or we may take our part
With brush or sculptor's knife,
And celebrate with work of art
God's feast of life.

(5) The God of Jesus praise,
The God who's yours and mine,
Who guides us through earth's teasing maze
Through cloud and shine.
We shall meet up at last
With Mary, John and Paul;
Jesus will proudly introduce us
- one and all!

(After Thomas Olivers 1725-99. Sung to Hebrew melody Leoni.)

Chapter Eight

HOITY TOITY.

One day when we were on our way to the same meeting place, we met a fortune-teller who used a large snake to pass on her messages. She was exploited by her employers, who made a lot of money out of her. She started following Paul and our team, shouting, "These people belong to the greatest God of all! They have a life-giving message for us!" She made a nuisance of herself like this for several days, until Paul became quite annoyed. At last he turned round and said, "You're sick! Jesus, God's Chosen, is going to make you better!" She was a new person from that moment on.

But when the girl's employers found they had lost their means of making money, they grabbed hold of Paul and Silas, and dragged them to the town hall. They made a complaint to the magistrates and said, 'These Jews are causing trouble in our town. The things they're telling us to do are against our Roman laws." The crowd started to get nasty, so the magistrates ordered Paul and Silas to be stripped and flogged. They got a bad beating and then they were put in prison. The warder was given special instructions to keep an eye on them. So he put them in a maximum security unit and chained them to the floor.

In the middle of the night Paul and Silas talked with God and sang songs. The other prisoners could hear it all. Suddenly there was a violent earthquake, which shook the foundations of the prison. Doors came off their hinges and the prisoners' chains were loosened. The warder woke up with a start, and when he saw the prison doors wide open, he grabbed his sword to kill himself. He thought the prisoners had escaped. But Paul yelled out to him, "Don't hurt yourself! We're all here!" The warder had the lights put on, and in a state of shock, ran into the cell and fell down shaking in front of Silas and Paul. Then he brought them out and asked them, "How can I learn to cope with life, like you?" They told him, "Put your trust in Jesus, and you will know true health and happiness, and so will the others in your house." Paul and Silas then gave God's message to the warder and the people who lived with him. It was still night when the warder washed their wounds. Without waiting for the morning, he and all his family were dipped. He took Paul and Silas into his house and gave them a meal. Everyone in the house was very excited and happy because the warder had put his trust in God.

In the morning the magistrates sent the police to the prison. They said, "You had better let those two prisoners go." The warder went to tell Paul. "The magistrates have sent to say you're free to go. They're dropping the charges." But Paul said, "They're not going to get away with this! They've beaten us in public and sent us to prison, all without a trial. You can't treat Roman citizens like that! If they think they're going to hush it all up, they can think again! Let them come and fetch us!" The police took this message back to the magistrates, who had a fright when they learned that Paul and Silas were Roman citizens. So they came to the prison and apologized. They gave them an escort out of the prison, and then requested them to leave the town. After their release from prison, Paul and Silas went back to Lydia's. They met their Christian sisters and brothers again, and put them in good heart. Then they left Philiptown.

2 Luke 16 (Acts): 16-40

A trouble-maker turned up at the smart church. I call the church 'smart' firstly because the people there look smart – suits and ties mostly for the men, hats or 'hairdos' for the ladies, almost without exception, and a gentle mixture of perfume and after-shave mingling with the tasteful floral decorations. The members have all been well-brought-up. They are pleasant to one another and look after one another when the need arises. They speak nicely and try to avoid contention. They give a lot of money to the missionary society and to charitable causes. They are inclined to the view that theirs is a 'good' church. It has a worthy history. It has had some notable ministers. Their pulpit has often been a springboard to further advancement. The attendance, though not what it used to be, has not yet gone down sufficiently to that point where it could be called 'thin'. There has been no need to engage in gimmicky evangelistic crusades or to introduce choruses in order to replenish the well-polished pews. There is a tradition of doing everything in order and good taste. Although it is rarely put into words or written down in a creed, the belief is implicit that the function of the church is to set an example to society as to how society at large should conduct itself. Occasionally a divorce among the members is an embarrassment and the aim when this happens is damage limitation, especially to the reputation of the church and Christian 'standards'. (As in most churches, because it is not supposed to happen, there is little in the way of teaching as to how the coming to an end of partner-ships can be approached in a constructive, Christian way.) 'Law and Order' feature highly among their political concerns, and many are Conservative voters of the more traditional true blue kind. Among their number are local dignitaries, magistrates and members of the police. It was definitely not the place for a 'trouble-maker' to do his turn. He was after help in the form of money, and when he failed to achieve his object, he became abusive. One of the church officers who was also a magistrate stepped in at this stage. "Leave this to me. We know how to deal with this type on the bench!" He showed the trouble-maker a seat and asked him to wait. The trouble-maker assumed he was going to fetch some money. When he returned it was in the company of a policeman. The trouble-maker obliged by giving more trouble in the way of abuse and lack of cooperation and the policeman was able to arrest him and bang him up in a police cell for the night. The church had had an unpleasant experience. What a blessing that it had among its members a man of stature with the experience of coping with this kind of character, and was in a position to arrange that conditions of bail would include a ban on his entering that church again! What a relief!

Paul was a Roman citizen. It was a status of which he was constantly aware and which he frequently reminded others of when it suited his purposes. Paul was strangely schizo when it came to a matter of privilege. He was prepared to count all his privileges as 'rubbish' compared with the privilege of knowing Jesus. But for someone who claimed to have made this extreme choice, he was inclined to harp on the privileges he had vowed to cast aside rather often. Yes, he had given all up for Jesus, but we are not to forget that he was a 'Hebrew of the Hebrews' – those entrusted with the privilege of bearing the God's messages, nor that he was a pupil of Liam, nor that he had had the opportunity of arriving at an appreciation of Greek culture, nor that he had the necessary skills to earn his own keep and not depend on the charity of others, and above all that he was not, like so many of his contemporary Christians, a slave or something close, but 'free-born', a citizen of the Roman Empire with all the rights and privileges that went with it.

Paul's Roman citizenship was undoubtedly the key whereby he was able to approach important Roman officials like George Paul with a view to their conversion. It also enabled him to extricate himself on occasions from difficult situations, for example when he was arrested in Jerusalem and avoided a flogging on the strength of his status. (GAN 287) He escaped trial by his own Jewish people by appealing to the Emperor, as was his right. (GAN 291) The policy of converting members of the Roman officialdom was a wise one. It gave the Jesus people friends in high places. It also assured others that the new religion was consistent with civil obedience and that Christians were not out to cause the breakdown of society. This is reflected in Paul's letter to Rome, chapter 13, where Paul puts the stamp of God's approval on stable government as part of the good order God has planned for the world. (GAN 320) (This passage received a heavily biased translation in the 1611 'authorized' English version with a view to pleasing James I with his 'divine right of kings'.) Paul's teaching here can only be understood in the light of the debt he owed to his place within the Roman order. There must have been many a first century Christian suffering for want of Paul's special protection who would not have put it quite like Paul. We do not have their views in writing apart perhaps from the coded outcries in the harsh and bitter Book of Revelation.

On one occasion Paul's use of his Roman citizenship was very curious. At Philiptown he and Silas were arrested, beaten and thrown into prison. It was to be the scenario for the conversion of the prison warder, one of the most exciting stories in Luke's second volume. Paul and Silas kept the other prisoners awake by singing songs, and an earthquake opened up the prison, causing the warder to make a dramatic gesture towards suicide. Paul and Silas were seen in a different light when they answered for the safety of the other prisoners. What the other prisoners thought of this we are not told! The reversal of fortunes was sealed when the magistrates ordered that Paul and Silas be released. It is at this point that Paul chose to reveal that both of them were Roman citizens and had therefore been dealt with illegally. Paul demanded an official escort out of the prison in order, we presume, to make the apology public, and, it would seem, to cause embarrassment.

They're not going to get away with this! They've beaten us in public and sent us to prison, all without a trial. You can't treat Roman citizens like that! If they think they're going to hush it all up, they can think again! Let them come and fetch us!

What was Paul playing at? Was there no point previously, when he was being arrested, when prepared for flogging, or put in the irons, that he could not have made known his citizenship? A 'spiritual' interpretation may be that the Spirit prompted Paul to silence in order to make the opportunity for converting Clem, the prison warder, who was to be the first male member in the (at first) all female Philiptown Christian community. Clem doubtless provided invaluable assistance to Lydia, the leader. But there is always something fishy about the calculated suppression of truth and it is difficult to fit 'the Spirit of Truth' into such an explanation. It looks much more like a careful ruse on Paul's part to use his status to maximum effect and to give the maximum amount of discomfort to his persecutors – 'heaping coals of fire on their heads', translated in Good As New as 'That will give them something to think about!" (pg.320)

The magistrates were impressed and duly provided the requested escort. But we are not told that they were converted, and that's hardly surprising. An even more bizarre thought, but none-the-less difficult to avoid, is that Paul and Silas indulged in a spot of masochism, allowing themselves to be beaten when they could have avoided it. Suffering for the truth is one thing, suffering in order to put yourself in an invincible position of moral superiority is something else. The closeness Paul and Silas achieve with Clem and his family as they seek spiritual enlightenment contrasts unfavorably with the uneasy deference provided by the blushing magistrates. They were glad to see them on their way. Paul was such a mixture. So warm and affectionate at times, so defensive and paranoid at other times; so reliant on God's grace at one point, so proud of externals at the next. At Philiptown he over used and manipulated a privilege that for a follower of Jesus should have counted for little. He was acting the 'drama queen', he was being HOITY TOITY!

Luke's opinion? No glimmer of disapproval can be detected with any certainty, unless the interpretation I have given of Paul's behavior is deducible from the way Luke tells the story. If he had wanted to make things look better for Paul he could have recorded the escort without reporting Paul's demand for it. That would have looked impressive and would have only been an abbreviation, not a bending of the truth. We would like to say to Luke, "As you wrote about the special escort given to Paul as a

Roman citizen, did you recall the disapproval of Jesus of those who sought places of honor? (1Luke 11:43; 14:7 & 20:26) Was Paul's behavior different in kind from the members of the strict set, the Pharisees, who liked to be on display, cherished their privileges and who insisted on the best places at dinner?

Hoity-toity behavior creates barriers. It does not produce the respect it is calculated to obtain. It makes affection very difficult, unless you know the person well enough to make allowances, which the Philiptown magistrates did not in the case of Paul. The trouble-maker who entered the church was looking for money and also for acceptance as a human being, and perhaps, with slim hope, for affection. He got a demonstration of strength and cunning and of the ability of privilege to put others down. If the church concerned ever reads this chapter they will not recognize themselves or will say it wasn't really like that. See yourselves as others see you, people of God! See yourself as those you humiliated at Philiptown see you, Paul! Then you will remember your words about not boasting, save in Christ! (e.g. GAN 390)

There is more than one way of being 'hoity-toity'. When I was a student at Southampton I used to pass on my way to evening worship on Sundays a little group of Christians who held a service on a street corner. They seemed to take turns for one of their number each week to address the passers-by. I felt very sorry for them, for apart from myself and a few other church-goers, no one took any notice of them. It would have been surprising if a passer-by managed to catch a whole sentence, let alone follow the intricacies of the Pauline theology being presented. The opportunity came for me to have a chat with one of their number. I asked him if he ever became discouraged in view of the lack of response to his ministry. He said, "I don't think about it. I preach the message. If people don't want to hear it, that's their lookout!"

The attitude of the street-corner evangelist is poles apart from the attitude of Jesus as he proclaimed the good news. The good news was that God cared for people with a love that exceeds that of the best earthly parent. The authenticity of this love finds proof both in the way Jesus presented his message in the context of care for all the needs and concerns of his hearers, and in the way he was wounded when it was rejected. Nowhere did Jesus find so bitter a rejection than in the big city. But love does not shrug its shoulders. As Jesus, with horror, contemplated the fate of Jerusalem, he wept bitterly. (GAN 227) His sense of loss was comparable to the sense of loss at losing a dear friend. The cross was the clearest sign of rejection of Jesus by those he came to help. It was also the place where love made its most amazing response. "Forgive them, Loving God! They don't know what they are doing!"

Unrequited love has many ways of coping. Romantics write poetry and get it out of their system. Some look for time to heal. Others rationalize – "There are plenty more fish in the sea." God bears the pain and goes on to show even more proof of love.

In his second volume, Luke records the response of Paul's rejection by his own compatriots in Corinth. (GAN 278) Paul demonstrates a similar attitude to our street-corner 'evangelist'. In line with his usual way of operating, he began his mission in Corinth by addressing first the people of the synagogue. But when on this occasion they proved difficult, Paul shook the dust from his clothes and said, "I've had enough of you. You're on your own from now on. It's other peoples' turn!" To be fair to Paul, these were not always his feelings when he contemplated the rejection of the good news by his own people. What happened in Corinth was an outbreak of frustration and impatience in the heat of the moment. When writing to the Jesus community at Rome, Paul had time to reflect, and he wrote, "So strong are my feelings for my own people, the Jews, that I would forfeit my own lifeline with Jesus, if by so doing they could experience his new life." (GAN 314) That's better, Paul! Paul, the mixture again – so conformed to the mind of Jesus on some occasions, so much a prey to his less lovely emotions on others.

The question of responsibility is a tricky one. How responsible are we for those we feel under the obligation to pass on the good news? It seems so reasonable a notion that providing we have done all we can to help somebody else, then, if they fail to do their part, our responsibility is at an end. I've attempted to sort this one out as a teacher, but not entirely to the satisfaction of my peace of mind. I still pass or fail with my pupils. The Good News has to do with an offer of love, and the responsibilities of love never come to an end. Even at its most helpless love watches and waits and has ways of making itself known. As Paul's better self knew very well, "...love sticks at it and never admits defeat." (GAN 345)

Possibly Paul's behavior towards the Jews at Corinth derived from the advice given by Jesus to the friends he sent out as missionaries. Good As New records his words like this: "If you get a bad reception, hold a peaceful demonstration in the street, and say, 'We're going on our way, because you have not made us feel at home. Even so, we leave you this message, "God's New World has come near to you today." ' (GAN 205) This peaceful demonstration will, literally, involve the friends wiping off the dust of the inhospitable town from their feet. This action seems rude to us, but it had more to do with the preservation of dignity. The situation anticipated by Jesus was somewhat different from that which Paul encountered in Corinth. Just as Jesus advised the acceptance of whatever food was put in front of the friends, kosher or non-kosher, as a sign of hospitality graciously given, so the shaking off the dust was a to be a sign of hospitality ungraciously refused. The message would not at this stage have been preached, accepted or rejected. But far from absolving the missionaries from responsibility if they failed to be welcomed with smiles, they were to proclaim the good news as they departed. God's New World is near and that is good news for everybody no matter whether or not the messengers find acceptance. The question of hospitality is another matter and has to do with customs of politeness and good manners in eastern societies. Those who flout the accepted basic human decencies are behaving like Sodom of old. That was a long time previous and the peoples of the Middle East had had time to improve their manners since then. So Jesus, with a wince, says that Sodom will do better in the performance league tables than those who were inhospitable in his day.

In contrast, at Corinth, Paul publicly resigned his responsibility towards his own people. Whereas the friends sent out by Jesus were told to withdraw with dignity when rejected, Paul's behavior comes across as pique. He was being hoity-toity again.

Followers of Jesus should avoid hoity-toity behavior. People are free to take to us or otherwise. If they don't take to us it is not always possible to assess the reasons why. It may be them; it may be us; it may be circumstances. We have a battery of weapons at hand if we choose to be vindictive, not least the ability to wipe our memory clean of them. Love in advance and love in retreat is the way of Jesus.

Those who are down

(1) Those who are down need fear no fall,
Those who are low no pride;
Those who are humble always will
Have God close by their side.

(2) Let's be content with what we have,
Unless it is too much;
Then we should try to shed the load
Lest conscience lose its touch.

(3) "Carry no pack", our Leader said;
"Whether of goods or care.
My venture will full strength require,
Joy is for those who dare."

(4) Jesus, life was for you so rough,
Yet you found ease of mind;
Teach us the secret in our day
When peace is hard to find,

(5) Help us to mind not what we lose
Or what we fail to gain,
Give thanks for comforts real and not
Make too much of our pain.

(6) Thank you for giving each our cross;
We could not shoulder yours;
As someone helped you bear its weight,
You gladly help with ours.

(7) Those who are down need fear no fall;
You greet them, "Come on up!"
Those who are humble sit, amazed,
To share your food and cup.

(After John Bunyan 1628-88 Tune: Arden or St, Bernard)

Chapter Nine

OTHER TONGUES.

It was the spring holiday, and they were all there.It was just like a hurricane sweeping out of the sky. You could hear the noise all over the house. Sudden streaks of light darted about and lit up one friend after the other. They were all filled by God's Spirit, and she gave them the ability to communicate in new ways.

There were many Jews staying in Jerusalem at that time, from every country in the known world. The noise attracted a big crowd. It was strange that, though they had different languages, they could all understand what the friends were saying. They found it incredible and said, "They're ordinary working people from Galilee! How can they communicate with us? They're talking about the exciting things God has been doing, and we can understand every word, just as if we were hearing it in our own language!" (There were people there from the countries round the Persian Gulf and further east, from the Celtic lands, from North Africa, Arabia, Crete and Rome, as well as from districts nearby. Some had been born Jews, others were Jewish converts.) They were impressed and confused at the same time, anxious to know what it was all about. Some thought the whole thing funny and said, "It looks as if they've had a few drinks!"Luke Part Two (Acts) 2: 1-13.

Love is the talent you should be trying to develop. The other talents God's Spirit gives are worth having too, especially the ability to explain God's truth. The language some people use is so difficult, only God can understand it. If you know how to communicate, you can stimulate, encourage and comfort people. Those who use fancy language give themselves a treat, but those who give a clear message benefit the whole community. I would like all of you to have language skills, but getting the point across is even more important. The one who explains things, so that everyone understands, is more valuable to the community than the one who uses big words and long sentences, unless there is someone who can put what has been said in more simple terms afterwards.

So friends, what use is it if, when I come to see you, you can't understand a word I say? I can only help you if I make things clear, or give you some information or insight you can grasp immediately. Those of you who play musical instruments, like the flute or harp, will understand what I mean. If the tune is too complicated, people won't be able to sing along. Soldiers need to be able to recognize the tunes their trumpeters play, otherwise they'll misunderstand their orders. How can people expect to know what you're talking about if you don't use language they can understand? Your words will go in one ear and out the other! There are lots of different languages in the world, and they all mean something to somebody. But if I can't understand the words someone is using, and they can't understand me, it will be difficult for us to become friends. So if you're serious about developing a talent, choose a talent which is helpful to others.

Someone who uses language which is difficult to follow, must ask God for the ability to be simple. Sometimes when I'm talking with God I'm so wrapped up, I'm not aware of what I'm saying. Something that has nothing to do with my mind has taken over. What should I do about this? It's okay to get worked up and express your emotions when you talk with God. But you should keep a firm grip on your mind at the same time. Sing heartily, by all means, but think carefully about what you're singing. If you're speaking words of thanks to God, how can visitors to your meeting respond by shouting their agreement, if they don't know what you're talking about? It's no good making what you consider to be a fine speech if other people can't understand you. I owe it to God that I can speak more languages than any of you. But when I'm in a meeting with other Christians, I'd sooner speak a few carefully-thought-out words, so the others who are there learn something, than babble on at great length in a language no-one can understand!

Don't be childish, dear friends. It's good to have a childlike innocence. But your thinking should be grown up. As the old books say,

'People of different tongues will speak
Truths to my people so proud;
But though it's done on my behalf,
They'll be deaf to every word.'

This shows the need to develop language skills for taking the good news to people of other cultures, whereas the ability to explain God's truth in greater depth is needed for the benefit of those who are already Christians. If when you meet together everyone is spouting off in different languages, visitors will think you very peculiar. But if everyone is out to explain some aspect of Christian truth, visitors will see where their lives have been going wrong. (If they don't take any notice, it will be their own fault.) They may come face to face with themselves for the first time in their lives. They may end up joining in the worship and say, "We know God is here with you!" '

First letter to Corinth 14: 1-1

Something very strange happened on the first Whitsunday that has never been adequately explained. We are told by Luke that the friends of Jesus were all filled with God's Spirit and started talking in 'other tongues' (traditional versions). Visitors from many parts of the world were able to understand what they said and this was a source of astonishment in view of the fact that the friends were Galileans, that is, uneducated country types. There may be a rational explanation of what happened. In teaching his disciples Jesus may have used the method of teaching 'by rote', and with foresight he may have provided them with an element of bilingualism, drilling them in a series of key phrases in one or both of the two common languages that would have been familiar to most pilgrims from the Greek world – traditional Hebrew or basic Greek. A real Devonian speaking the full Devonian dialect (now regrettably almost died out) would have a job to communicate with a Geordie from Tyneside. North Walians and South Walians who speak idiomatic Welsh sometimes have the same problem.

Neither the Devonian nor the Geordie has any difficulty in understanding a BBC commentator, and North Walians and South Walians can follow 'Newyddion' (the news in Welsh). There may also have been a degree of body language involved. In my culture our use of body language has become minimalized, though it is still there to the informed observer. In other cultures body language is much more pronounced and bears a much larger part in communication, especially where there are language difficulties. The age of television has brought about a rebirth of the skills of communicating visually. I was interested to find that Benny Hill was the most popular show with a group of Chinese students who were lodging with a friend of mine. The reason was that the story line could be followed with ease without any comprehension of the almost non-existent dialogue. Christian ministers these days try to communicate visually (often clumsily) with their overhead projectors and computer systems. They could learn a thing or two from Benny Hill! (Someone should perhaps tell the younger generation of preachers that no amount of sophisticated equipment can conceal the fact when they have nothing particular to say, and that there is no more effective way of getting a message across than the spoken word, if you know how to do it!)

Whatever the rational explanation of the tongues of Whitsunday, their meaning and purpose is very clear. The purpose was to communicate the 'Good News' of Jesus to those who otherwise would not have understood it. The meaning, which many commentators note, was a reversal of the story of the Tower of Babel (Genesis 11) where confusion of tongues is depicted as an aspect of disunity among the nations. On the Day of Pentecost God's Spirit broke down the barriers of language and made the unity of humanity a fresh possibility. Further on in Luke's second volume, we find conversion, dipping, and the gift of God's Spirit frequently accompanied by 'speaking in tongues', though not always. It is a pity we have no precise description of what on these occasions the gift of tongues involved. Were the tongues a means of communication as at Pentecost, and if so, from whom and to whom? Or were they just some kind of sign that the Spirit had been given? A ticket or passport to church membership? On at least one occasion the original Pentecost meaning of tongues was preserved. In the case of Neil, the Roman centurion, the gift of tongues seems to have been the deciding factor which convinced Rocky that a Gentile was eligible, as he was, to join the church without becoming a Jew. More importantly perhaps, Rocky used this piece of evidence to convince waverers and confound his critics. The need of Rocky and others to draw quickly on whatever arguments they could muster to get a hesitating church to broaden its outlook and extend its boundaries must be taken into account. The leaders often did not have the opportunity to reflect on the long-term consequences of the stratagems they employed. In that respect we must not be too hard on them. The point remains that in the case of Neil the Pentecost meaning of tongues held true, for it signaled the breaking down of barriers between cultures and indeed religions. Before Rocky's visit Neil was a worshipper of God, acceptable to God, though neither Jew nor Christian.

The next evidence we have of speaking in tongues comes from about twenty years later from Paul's letters to the Christian community in Corinth. This was a community with problems. The overall problem was disunity, and doubtless this was a matter of personalities, as is usually the case. Members were entering into competition with one another to show off their spiritual gifts, in particular the gift of 'tongues'. Tongues which at Pentecost was the symbol of unity, now appears as the cause of disunity. There are other differences. The whole point of the Whitsunday tongues was that they were understood. There would have been nothing to write home about otherwise! Tongues at Corinth were a meaningless 'gibberish' (Paul's word: 14: 11 REV) and needed an interpreter. Moreover, far from being the means of winning over the unbeliever, Paul is of the opinion that tongues would only put an unbeliever off. It looks very much as if somewhere between Whitsunday and Corinth the gift of tongues has been debased.

Tongue speaking is still a lively issue amongst Christians. The twentieth century saw the rapid growth of Pentecostalist churches, nearly all of whom practice speaking in tongues. The last half of that century saw the emergence of the 'Charismatic Movement' which touched nearly all denominations, including Catholics and Episcopalians. The movement emphasized the need to express the 'charisma', the gifts of the Spirit, the gift of tongues being one such gift.

The tongues spoken in Pentecostal churches and in charismatic groups appear to be those of Corinth and *not* those of Whitsunday. There have been few instances of Whitsunday tongue speaking since the first. In the fourteenth century Vincent Ferrer is said to have converted people all over Europe, speaking many different tongues and dialects, without apparently having had the opportunity to learn the languages. In the sixteenth century Louis Bertrand is said to have converted 300,000 indigenous people from various tribes and dialects in South America. Francis Xavier and Hildergard are also among the Catholic saints who were canonized on the basis of having this particular gift. Neither should it be forgotten that Francis of Assisi preached to the birds. Either this was an eccentric nonsense exercise or the birds understood by means of the Spirit. Francis at any rate appreciated the full significance of the text of Joel that the Spirit was intended for 'all flesh'. His precedent does not seem to have been widely copied. More recent instances of real communication through an unlearnt unfamiliar tongue are few and far between and not very convincing.

I hazard the unexciting opinion that the modern equivalent to the Whitsunday experience is a missionary getting down to her books and language CDs and learning to speak a new language properly, and doing this hand in hand with an in-depth appreciation of the cultural background of the language, which is just as important for true communication to take place as a knowledge of the language itself. Another parallel, even less exciting for those who are out to get quick thrills, is the on-going task of re-interpreting the faith, together with the scriptures, as history moves on and culture develops and changes. Perhaps we have done a little Whitsunday speaking in tongues in 'Good As New'.

What then of those who speak in tongues Corinth style? They fall into three main categories. There are those who believe tongues of this kind to be essential to Christian experience. This runs totally against the teaching of Paul in his first letter to Corinth. In his well-known description of the body of Christ, just as the different parts or members of the body have different functions, so the gifts of the Spirit are distributed throughout the Christian community. Paul asks,

God wants everyone to count – leaders, speakers, teachers, artists, healers, administrators, enablers, and communicators. No one can do all those jobs at the same time! (12:29)

The second group, though they do not regard 'tongues' as essential to the Christian, nevertheless regard it as a super-plus. Tongue speaking is *the* proof of genuine spirituality. Again, such a view flies in the face of Paul's teaching. For Paul *love* is the supreme gift

I may be an impressive speaker, but if I haven't got love, my words will be like an unpleasant banging sound that gets on your nerves.(13:1)

The gift of tongues is also inferior to that of prophesy. (Prophesy in the Biblical sense does not mean clairvoyance, but speaking God's message clearly to the present situation.)

I would like all of you to have language skills, but getting the point

across is even more important. The one who explains things, so that everyone understands, is more valuable to the community than the one who uses big words and long sentences... (14:5)

Paul seeks to give a death blow to the idea that tongues are the means of being spiritually one-up.

I owe it to God that I can speak more languages than any of you. but when I'm meeting with other Christians, I'd sooner speak a few carefully thought-out words, so the others who are there can learn something, than babble on at great length in a language nobody can under-stand!(14:18)

The third group of tongue speakers make a genuine effort to follow the teaching of Paul on tongues. They accept tongues as a true gift of the Spirit, but use it with restraint, normally in private or in the company of believers where an interpreter must be present. There can be little quarrel on any grounds with this shade of opinion. Even if it is difficult to see the point of such 'tongues', it is difficult to see any harm. But we cannot avoid the question of whether the revival of Corinthian tongues is appropriate to our times.

Paul claimed the gift of tongues. (It should not be forgotten that Paul was a good linguist, not the least of his qualifications as an ace missionary. He could probably speak Latin, Classical Hebrew, Greek and Aramaic competently at least, though not the early form of Welsh spoken by the Galatians. The gift of tongues failed him at Lester (Lystra)! – Luke Part Two (Acts) 14) But it seems he also had a go at Corinthian tongues, though he preferred not to do it in company, restricting the practice of it to his private devotions. He says,

Those who use fancy language give themselves a treat, but those who give a clear message benefit the whole community. (14:4)

Paul goes on to say:

Sometimes when I'm talking with God, I'm so wrapped up, I'm not aware of what I'm saying. Something that has nothing to do with my mind has taken over. What should I do about this? It's okay to get worked up and express your emotions when you talk with God. But you should keep a firm grip on your mind at the same time. (14: 13)

Paul seems to be trying to get his head around a practice the first Christians have somehow landed themselves with and which will not go away. We can imagine that privately he values 'tongues' even less than he is prepared to admit in his letter. He is building bridges with those for whom tongues has become important, even an obsession. In private devotions when words fail to match feelings, then the use of inarticulate noises may be one way of relieving the tension. Others may find quiet, deep breathing, yoga exercises, their way of achieving the same end. The noisy form of release, or spiritual buzz, seems to be what Paul is talking about when in another letter he says,

The Spirit is a big help when we're finding it hard to cope. Sometimes it's difficult to put our feelings into words to God. That's where the Spirit comes in. She interprets the deep desires we can only express as groans.(Letter to Rome 8: 26)

Some psychiatrists believe 'tongues' to be a form of release for unresolved emotional conflicts and thus therapeutic. This accords with the evidence from charismatic groups of people cured of anti-social behavior through tongue-speaking. Carl Gustav Jung made a study of the phenomenon and thought tongues to be a window into an inherited communal consciousness. We must not close our minds.

An inclusive Christianity may have to follow Paul's line and find a place for something many do not have an inclination to be enthusiastic about. But any values tongues may be found to have will need constantly to be checked against the dangers of spiritual pride, giving offence to others and creating further divisions. The Christian community at Corinth was not a happy one, despite everybody going for tongues, hell-for-leather.

We need to take careful note of the marked difference between Whitsunday tongues and Corinthian tongues. This means accepting that within the 'apostolic' period, at the very time the Church was under the leadership of Rocky, Paul and James, Jesus' brother, there was a debasement in both the practice and the understanding of an important feature of the Good News. Whatever value Corinthian tongues may have, they are not Whitsunday tongues. The Charismatic Movement can be seen as a protest against the intellectualizing of Christianity. By compromising with the rationalism of the late nineteenth and early twentieth centuries we have forgotten the use the Spirit can make of our emotions and our bodies. This should be an argument for adjusting the balance, not for despising the intellect. For Paul, inspiration and intelligence are not opposites. They are meant to go hand in hand.

Sing heartily, by all means, but think carefully about what you're singing.(14:15)

On that basis, a large number of our so-called charismatic choruses wouldn't stand a chance! I'm always amused and concerned to read at the beginning of the chorus 'Abba Father' the words, 'Sing thoughtfully'. If we sang thoughtfully we would fall silent after the first two lines. *'Let me be yours and yours alone?'* – impossible and not at all what God wants. A moment's thought would put us right.

Much of our liturgical material would not pass Paul's test. It is a form of speaking in tongues in the sense that very few, if any, can understand it. But, especially if it is ancient, it gives us a warm and holy glow. Paul would tell us to chuck it.

Our times have presented the faith with an intellectual challenge. If we run away from that challenge, the Christian church will eventually end up as one of many occult oddities, of interest only to dabblers. Whitsunday was not the first occasion of soaking in the Spirit. Jesus received the Spirit when he was dipped by John in the River Jordan. There is no suggestion that Jesus spoke in tongues Corinthian style. He spoke in tongues Whitsunday style. The teacher who could hold ordinary people spell-bound for a whole day in a dry, hot desert, had the gift of tongues. His appeal was popular, and at the same time offered no insult to the highest intelligences of his day.

Now we must come to the question of the apostles' responsibility for the debasement of the gift of tongues. Without a doubt, much in the early Christian communities was out of the apostles' control, and we should perhaps be grateful for that. If the future direction of the Church had been in the hands of Rocky and Lightning (John), or even of Paul, much of the spontaneity we confidently call the leading of the Spirit would have been lacking. The break with Temple worship and the restrictions of the Jewish Law, the Gentile Mission, the progress of the Good News among Roman officialdom, and so on, were things that came about very largely from pressure outside the apostolic circle. At the same time the apostles were a direct link to the mind of Jesus, though there may always have been others who knew that mind better. The apostles had the responsibility to put a hand on the tiller if the ship strayed too far from the course they believed Jesus had set it on. Although there is foundation in the ministry of Jesus for Whitsunday tongues, properly understood as the use and development of communication skills, there is nothing that can be detected as the basis of Corinthian tongue speaking. The nearest perhaps is Jesus at the graveside of Larry (Lazarus) the 'Beloved Disciple' when, according to the Greek words used, Jesus expressed his anguish in sounds that resembled the howling of a dog, the roaring of a bull and the croaking of a frog. That was close, perhaps, to Paul's groaning in his private devotions, but nothing to do with the spiritual showing off that went on in Corinth. What seems to have happened is that the skills in which Jesus groomed his friends, and which they had the confidence to use on the Day of Pentecost, quickly became something quite different. Tongues became a fetish. In a period when there must have been much anxiety and questioning as to who was a true Christian and who was not, the litmus test became the possession of the Spirit, and this was most quickly and conveniently demonstrated by the production of 'tongues'.

Were there no doubts and hesitations among the friends of Jesus as new converts obediently spouted the required amount of gobbledygook? Provided that one or two words, foreign or otherwise, could be detected, hey-presto they had the gift? As long as somebody standing by said they understood it, then the novices passed the test? Sounds like the emperor's clothes! What on earth were the apostles thinking about to allow a situation like this to develop? Convenient or otherwise to have some kind of test over which they could and did act as inspectors, how could they justify it from the teaching of the Leader? According to the parable of Jesus recorded in Matthew, and which the gospel writer is probably using to provide direction for the Christian communities, although someone sows weeds among the harvest, it is not possible to tear up the weeds until harvest time, since pulling up the weeds would involve pulling up the crop. Both must be left until harvest. (13:24) The Church cannot anticipate God's judgment by picking and choosing who it will have on its territory. The parable of the sheep and the goats makes the same point. Out on the mountain-side sheep and goats are just specks, difficult to distinguish from one another. Only when they are rounded up and penned at the end of the day can they be told apart. (Matthew 25). By using the gift of tongues in the way they did, the apostles were treading very dangerous ground. Not only did they set a test that could exclude, as and when they thought fit, but they opened the floodgate to religiosity – their teacher's enemy number one. Once it had been established that someone who demonstrated tongues had the Spirit, it was going to be difficult to prevent that person from taking on airs.

What keeping the law in an exemplary manner did for the Strict Set (The Pharisees), tongues did for the first Christians, as Paul in his first letter to Corinth makes clear. 'Working wonders' or healing the sick or a degree of accurate future-telling would do as well as tongue speaking for test purposes, but tongues was by far the easiest sign to produce at the drop of a hat, and also the easiest to fake. The other disaster brought about by the use of tongues as a test of the Spirit was to limit an understanding of the presence of the Spirit, if not to tongues alone, then to tongues and other similarly exciting phenomena. The Spirit was to be looked for in the extraordinary and peculiar even, and therefore missed elsewhere. This again was something Paul set his mind to tackling in Corinth. He was, in large measure, endeavoring to counter an inadequate doctrine and practice of the spirit that his fellow apostles had done much to encourage.

Did Luke share the reservations of his friend Paul with regard to tongue speaking? We cannot really tell from his descriptions in his second volume. He may be just giving us a dispassionate account of what happened among the first Christians. But it looks more as if he enters into the excitement of those early days, suspending to a degree his critical faculty. As far as Luke's judgment is concerned, he would have been greatly influenced by the role that tongue speaking played in the acceptance of non-Jews into the Christian community, being of Greek origin himself. If tongue speaking had its down-side, it certainly could boast the household of Neil, a high ranking Roman army officer, as a positive achievement.

However, Luke does not always mention the gift of tongues when he describes the coming of the Spirit. When Rocky and

Lightning 'correct' the work of Philip in Samaria and the people there receive God's Spirit, there is no mention of tongues. When the Ethiopian is dipped, Luke does not even mention him receiving the Spirit. Philip is still doing things his own way, successfully. There are no tongues, but there is joy! Joy is the sign of the Spirit in the multi-ethnic Christian community in Antioch, (2Luke 13:52) and in the household of the jailer at Philiptown. (16: 34) No mention of tongues here, nor in the case of the important conversion of Lydia who is to be the leader of the Philiptown church. (16:11) Lydia is described as opening her mind. Would that the Spirit's gift of an open mind were more widespread in the Church today! There is no mention of the fortune teller with the talking python receiving the gift of tongues, though she was already a good ventriloquist. Paul, in his letter to Philiptown, was not obliged to tell his friends in that town to retrain their outbursts of pious piffle. They were a calm and sensible lot.

Either Luke means us to assume in these cases that the Spirit is given in the usual way, with tongue speaking, or he is doing his best to play that aspect down. It is an important issue again in Ephesus, where Paul came across some 'disciples' who had not even heard of the Spirit. (19:2) These people seem to have been disciples of John the Dipper who probably still had a following separate from that of Jesus at that time. Paul decided that the right thing to do was to dip them again, this time in the name of Jesus. This is debatably a 'bad act'. Paul seems to be putting a very un-Pauline emphasis on an outward action. He is also giving the green light to the idea that if any baptism is deemed to have been inadequate, there is a case for a re-baptism. Most Baptists would agree with Paul on this one, though they would insist that in such circumstances the wishes of the individual concerned should be taken into account. Critics of the Baptist position are liable to feel uneasy and to point out that the circumstances were exceptional. Paul was not out to create a precedent. There is perhaps a parallel with Neil's household in that tongues are again brought out for special display to ratify the inclusion of another previously excluded section into the Christian community.

So then, Luke's view of tongue speaking is difficult to gauge. My guess is that he was less enthusiastic about it than were the people he described as doing it, and that as his story proceeds he looks for other less dramatic evidences of the Spirit, such as wisdom or joy. Paul, following the life and example of Jesus, believes the chief evidence of the Spirit is love, though he and the other apostles bear some of the responsibility for putting us off the scent.

'LOVE ALONE'

With great pleasure and appreciation I have added this 'polished' version of the Apostle Paul's great hymn of love to my set of 'Buttons Polished' – hymns updated to enable them to be sung with honesty and enthusiasm in the twenty-first century. Stephen Best wrote the words for the celebration of his civil partnership and blessing together with his partner Paul at City United Reformed Church 5 May 2006. Valerie and I were privileged to be present as invited guests. As with my own polished buttons there are no copyright rules. Acknowledgement of Stephen's authorship is appreciated.

Any words which I may utter
Without love to reach their goal
Are no more than clashing cymbals
Empty gongs without a soul.
Though I conjure future visions,
Understand life's wherewithal,
And have faith which moves the mountains,
Without love I am not whole.

Acts of charitable giving
And the self-denial call,
If such actions have no loving,
I gain nothing from them all.
Love is patient, love is kindness,
Knows no envy, does not boast,
Bends itself to other's pathways,
Hopes, believes and endures all.

Everything has its own season,
Once a child, I now stand tall.
Though an adult, yet my vision
Through dark mirrors captures all.
While I search for understanding,
Faith and hope and love still call;
And in future generations
Love alone will outlive all.

Stephen Best 2006.(Tune: Blaenwern, or tune to similar meter)

Chapter Ten

LUCKY FALL

We caught the boat from Philiptown just after Easter. The boat took five days to get to Troy where the others were waiting. We stayed in Troy for a week.

On Sunday, when we met to share food together, Paul gave us a talk. This was because he was thinking of leaving the next day. Paul was still talking at midnight. The room upstairs where we were meeting was lit by a large number of oil lamps. A young man was sitting on the window ledge. He began to feel drowsy as Paul went on and on. Then he went right off to sleep and fell out of the window, down three floors. When his friends got to him they thought he was dead. But Paul came down, put his arms round him and hugged him tight. "Nothing to be worried about," Paul said, "He's still alive!" Paul led everybody back upstairs. Then he broke the bread and ate with those who were there. Afterwards he chatted with them till morning. Then Paul left the house. The young man, whose name in Greek* means 'a lucky fall', was taken home none the worse for his experience, and everybody was very relieved. (2Luke 20 6-12;*Eutychus)

The Christian community at Troy was meeting to celebrate the Jesus Meal. The atmosphere was solemn. For a start, the presiding 'apostle' liked it that way. He had had experiences of these celebrations getting out of hand, especially in Corinth, just across the water. There the Christians had gone over the top, some of them over-indulging their appetites in food and drink, while poorer members of the congregation who had come looking for a cheap bite were left to go hungry. Others abused the feast by indulging in jealous rivalries. So Paul decided that it would be better if Christians concentrated their attentions in the meal on a simple action of breaking a loaf of bread and drinking from a common cup, and that all other eating and drinking be done at home. To rub it in, he suggested that friends of Jesus centre their thoughts on the night Jesus was betrayed and remembered his death. This, Paul hoped, would sober things up. Probably he took the same line at Troy as he did with the Corinthians. This might even have been the occasion on which he introduced his new format for communion to the folk at Troy. To add to the solemnity, both Paul and the assembled friends had a strong instinct that this would be the last such meal they would have together. There is an uncanny resemblance to the 'last supper' Jesus had with his followers in the upstairs function room in Jerusalem. Paul, like his leader, was making for the Holy City, and there, like his leader, he would be arrested, never to be free to visit the churches again. To cap it all, the meeting took place in a room upstairs. Certainly it seems to have been far from the over-jolly occasions at Corinth which had given Paul such concern.

The Supper at Troy was preceded by a sermon. The proclamation of the Good News of Jesus and the Jesus Meal go hand in hand- the appeal to the mind through the spoken words, and the appeal to the senses of vision, touch and smell through the handling and the sharing of food and drink. However, Paul made a mistake. He preached for too long. At least one member of the congregation thought so, and that is probably one too many. He was a young man and he was sitting on the edge in two ways. He was at the edge of the group, which probably means he was an enquirer rather than a regular member of the group, and he was sitting on the edge of the open window.

Paul should have known better. He was well aware that preaching was not his special gift. In his second letter to the Christians at Corinth, he mentions the general view of his preaching skills:

I know what people say, "Paul writes great letters, full of

punch. But he's not much to look at, and a hopeless speaker!"
(GAN 2.Cor: 1:12 trad. 10:10)

Not everybody has the same gift. This was something Paul appreciated and he counseled other Christians to make sure they had a gift before they tried to use it.

By authority of the grace God has given me I say to everyone among you: do not think too highly of yourself, but form a sober estimate based on the measure of faith that God has dealt to each of you...Let us use the <u>different</u> gifts allotted to each of us by God's grace:*(Rom 12: 3&6 REV)*

I remember my college principal, who could be cruel, telling a student who he felt unlikely to become even a passable preacher – "Choose five hymns – long ones – and preach for no more than ten minutes!"(Baptists in those days were used to a sermon of at least half an hour!) Unkind to the student, but kind to future congregations if the advice were taken. Paul knew his limitations, but on this occasion, perhaps because of the emotional situation, he was out of control. He started at sundown and was still going on at midnight!

The young man fell asleep and fell out of the window. We are not told how many others nodded off, more safely and comfortably seated. Luke, bless him, spares Paul's blushes by recording that there were many oil lamps burning in that upstairs room to account for feelings of drowsiness. Paul broke off the sermon and went downstairs to give the young man the kiss of life.

The Good News is not supposed to send anyone to sleep, at least not by reason of its content or presentation. I sometimes reassure people who look tired and weary that the message of God's love and care is the best possible relaxant and that if they fall asleep as a result of hearing it they may be counted as living proof of its effectiveness. But the Good News is never boring. Jesus said, **"I want you to have a life packed with good things."** *(John 10:10 GAN)*

Those words of Jesus should form the basis of everything the friends of Jesus do in his name. I'm afraid there is still the view around, even more common when I was a youngster, that if it didn't hurt it wasn't good for you, and that if you enjoyed it, it was probably bad. The use of trendy gimmicks to make presentations more interesting is still regarded by some with great suspicion, and humor frowned on.

In the twentieth century there were two great movements of the Spirit that served to heighten interest in worship. The first was the Liturgical Movement in which those responsible for worship in the mainstream denominations set themselves to renew worship by making use of the best traditions of the church, from times long past and more recent. Its enthusiasts sought to increase the visual element in worship and to involve the congregation much more. Stephen Winward was the high priest for the Baptist churches in England especially. I mention his name, for he was a great soul and a great teacher and his work deserves to be remembered. He was sowing on very stony ground as far as his own denomination was concerned, but some seed bore fruit. Leaders of his caliber with something extra special to offer are very rare in our churches today. I often disagreed with Stephen, but if nothing else he obliged our ministers to think about what they were doing in worship, me included. He did his best to keep things moving and not get stuck in a rut, always quick to pick up on a good suggestion wherever it might come from. He was never boring and his church was always full. The Liturgical Movement saw some of the free churches being treated to ministers wearing varieties of colorful vestments, responsive prayers and readings, a degree of liturgical topography (moving from one place to another to do this or that) and even on special occasions, candles. Many Catholic and Anglican churches saw their altar moved forward so that the president could stand behind it facing the congregation, and there was increased involvement by the laity in parts of the worship previously the preserve of the priest.

The other movement of the Spirit was the Charismatic Movement. It too sought to liven up worship, though in a different sort of way. Greater enthusiasm, more spontaneity, a greater use of our bodies – raising arms, clapping, dancing even – choruses, a wider variety of musical instruments, and the use of 'gifts' from among the congregation. Even in churches which would not regard themselves as charismatic, a more physical exchange of the peace, as well as more lively, catchy hymn tunes might be attributed to the influence of the movement. There should be no hesitation in attributing both movements to the Spirit of God. Where both have sometimes gone astray is when those ideas and practices intended to serve the churches have been allowed to become tyrants and freedom is stifled once more.

Back to the young man who fell out of the window. Luke thinks it important to tell us that he was a young man. There are those who think worship should be livened up for the sake of the young. Not so. Worship should be livened up for the sake of everybody! But a colorful and engaging liturgical pattern, or choruses triumphalist or soppy with instrumental backing, or a combination of the whole lot, will not of its own do the trick, except for those for whom worship is primarily entertainment. Then there is no difference between traditional and funky, classical or pop. It is simply a matter of choice along the lines of personal indulgence. The Trojan teenager fell asleep because what Paul was saying ceased to have any interest for him. No amount of experiment with forms of worship can cover the Church's irrelevance. By all means present the message in the most attractive way your imagination can devise. But make sure you have a message worth presenting. Otherwise there are going to be a lot of very disappointed people. How exciting that the visiting preacher for the day is going to use a projector screen to get our attention at sermon time. What a let down when what goes on the screen is nothing but a series of banalities.

The Church is not only frequently irrelevant to young people today, it is also irrelevant to those who share with the young a keen and active interest in the great issues of our times. The threats to the world's environment; exploitation and cruelty to animals; the quest for personal freedom; world hunger and poverty; the movements for equality of race and sex; the many movements for justice and peace. These things, when and if they are touched upon at all in our churches, are addressed in such a way that we are rumbled as not having considered the issues carefully or deeply. Too frequently we hope to get away with a mixture of platitude and prejudice. We are not listening to what is going on out there. We are not contributing to the debates in an informed and enlightened way.

Did Paul know the young man in his congregation? Was he aware of him in his telling place on the edge of things? Was he aware of his interests, his concerns, his aspirations, his anxieties? Paul does not seem to have taken much notice of him until he fell out of the window. That might have been too late. Luke tells us his name was 'Eutychus' which means 'a lucky fall'. This must have been a name or nickname he was given after the event –too much of a coincidence otherwise. More than likely it was the baptismal name he chose, which means we were right in the first place to identify him as an enquirer rather than already a member. So we must presume a happy ending for the story from the Christian community's point of view and another significant step in the progress of the Good News.

Luke, however, chooses to put his tongue in his cheek, to tell us that when the young man felt better again the Christians went back upstairs. For Paul to continue his sermon where he left off? They went back upstairs to break bread! One can almost feel the release of tension among the Trojan Christians, not only because the lad was alright, but because he had done them all a favor in bringing the sermon to an end. Perhaps Paul was reminded by the needs of Eutychus that deeds are more important than words, love more important that faith. Broken bread: broken lives: shared bread; shared lives: eaten bread; full lives. And then they chatted until daybreak. At last came the chance for Eutychus to ask questions and maybe tell Paul a thing or two – the chance to make the Good News live in a genuine encounter between mind and heart.

WALK BESIDE ME

(1) Walk beside me, friend and lover,
Till we make that better land;
Strength and weakness match each other;
Hold me, firm and tender hand.
Spread the table, spread the table-
We will share a banquet grand! (x2)

(2) Meet me at the spring of water
Pure and clean and sparkling too.
Dreams of cloud and fire and thunder
Vanish as I drink with you.
Fill the glasses, fill the glasses,
We will drink to love and joy. (x2)

(3) When we reach that chilly river
Conquer my anxiety.
You are life, - and death's destroyer;
I will share your victory.
Keep me singing, keep me singing,
Now and to eternity. (x2)

(After William Williams Pantycelyn. Tune: 'Cwm Rhondda' John Hughes, Pontypridd)

Chapter Eleven

HIS BROTHER

The whole meeting was very quiet while Cheery and Paul talked about the remarkable things they and God had done together, with people who were not Jews. When they had finished, James, Jesus' brother, gave a summing up.

"Listen carefully, friends. Rocky has reminded us of the first occasion when God convinced us that non-Jews are alright to mix with, and that some of them belong to God already. This is in line with what God's speakers say in the old books.

'I'll come back again,' says God,
'The faith of David to restore.
This time it will be set to last,
And be an empty shell no more.
I want a larger family-
It's been my plan for many a year.
All nations will belong to me.'
God has no pets, that's very clear!

This is how I think we should approach this issue. We shouldn't make things difficult for non-Jews who are turning to God. We should write to them, asking them not to eat food which has come from dubious places; to behave responsibly in sexual matters; and not to eat meat which still has blood in it. That will do. Moses doesn't need any more supporters. His words are read every Saturday in all our places of worship."(2Luke (Acts) 15: 12-21).

Some years later:

The next day Paul visited James, Jesus' brother. The other leaders were there. After asking how they all were, Paul gave a complete account of the way peoples of all countries had responded to God through his efforts. When they heard this they thanked God. Then they said to Paul, "Friend, there are thousands of Jews here who've put their trust in Jesus. But they all believe in keeping the old rules and regulations. They've heard that you tell the Jews in other countries to forget all about Moses and not to cut the foreskins of their boys and other such customs. We don't really know what to do to prevent you having trouble from them. They're bound to find out you're here. What about this for an idea? Four of our men have grown their hair long because they're on special duties. If you sponsor these in the customary ceremony for bringing the special duties to an end, and if you pay for them to have their haircut, people will see that the rumors about you are false. They'll notice you joining in and keeping the rules. People of other nations who have become Christians are another matter. We sent them that letter we all agreed on, directing them not to buy food from the dubious places or to eat meat which has blood in it, and to behave responsibly in sexual matters." So next day, Paul acted as sponsor for the men. He went through all the special washings and went with them to the temple. He made the announcement that the special period had come to an end and that a gift would be made to God on behalf of each of the men.

These ceremonies lasted for a week. When they were almost through, some Jews from abroad who had recognized Paul in the worship center, called on the crowd of worshippers to get hold of him. They shouted, "Anyone who calls themselves a good Jew, come quickly and help. This is the man who goes everywhere slandering our people, telling them to throw away our rules and get rid of our center. Now to crown it all he's brought his stinking foreigners in here." (Someone had seen Paul in the city with Tommy, a friend from Ephesus, and made the mistake of thinking Paul had brought him into the center.) The commotion spread out into the city. People ran to see what was happening. Paul was taken hold of roughly and dragged out of the center. The doors were shut behind him. The crowd were out to beat Paul to death. But the commander in charge of the Roman soldiers was told there was rioting in Jerusalem. Quickly he brought a unit of soldiers with their officers to the trouble spot. When the rioters saw the commander with his soldiers, they took their hands off Paul. Then the commander arrested Paul, put handcuffs on him, and asked who he was and what he was up to. The people in the crowd were shouting several different things at once, making it impossible for the commander to make any sense of it. So he ordered Paul to be taken to the soldiers' barracks. When they came down the steps of the worship center, the pressure of the crowd was so strong, the soldiers had to carry Paul. The crowd followed all the way shouting, "Kill him."(21: 18- 36)

It can't have been easy having such a famous brother. Indeed all the evidence we have in the scriptures leads us to think that James did not get on particularly well with his elder brother Jesus, perhaps even resented his notoriety. About their early life together we can only imagine. It seems likely that Joseph, the skilled carpenter/mason of Nazareth, died before his family of at least seven children had grown up. Matthew tells us Jesus had four brothers, presumably named in order of age- James, Joseph, Simon and Jude, and also mentions sisters, meaning there must have been at least two. The only one of these we are to know anything about for anything approaching certainty is James. The veil of secrecy about the rest is rather surprising. As the eldest of the family and a male, Jesus would automatically have assumed the role of father. By that time, we must assume he was in his teens, had already learnt his father's trade as the eldest of the family did, and taken over the Nazareth shop, becoming bread winner for the family.

My late mother-in-law, Joyce Styles of Herne Bay Baptist, was a down-to-earth, loyal and loving Christian. She lost her mother through death when she was still a child. Joyce and her younger brothers were brought up by her elder sister. When over ninety years of age, she still showed resentment at what she perceived as the less than ideal efforts of her sister/foster mother. We must assume - it seems to fit- that Jesus did not leave home to pursue his calling as a missionary/teacher/healer until his brothers and sisters were old enough to cope without him. Possibly James and the others resented being told what to do by a substitute father. Be that as it may, they had difficulty in understanding Jesus. Jesus was a genius. Had there been such a thing as MENSA in his day, Jesus would have been eligible. At twelve, he could hold his own with the ace rabbis in the temple at Jerusalem. Geniuses are usually odd, or rather appear odd to those around them. They are often lonely because it is difficult for them to find companions who can follow the pattern of their thought. James was not 'thick', as his later skilful and sensitive leadership of the Jerusalem Christian community was to prove. But intellectually he was not in the same league as his brother. The witness of scripture is that the family of Jesus at first did not sympathize with Jesus' ministry, neither his mother, his brothers or his sisters. That's very sad, since Jesus was the most sociable of people. He was to have a wide circle of friends from all classes of society. But he did not have a friend at home, nor an admirer even, it would seem. Whenever Jesus returned home he received a chilly welcome which led him on at least one occasion to remark, "It's strange how God's speakers are appreciated everywhere except where they come from and by their families!" (From a Jewish Friend 13:53 - Matthew)

'Sources Close' (John's Gospel) tells us another story that makes the same point about the relationship between Jesus and his family. Jesus was touring Galilee, not far away from home. His brothers came to see him and tried to persuade him to leave the district and go south to Jerusalem. Their argument was that Jerusalem was a better setting for someone wanting to be in the public eye. It looks as if they thought their brother was nothing but an attention-seeker. It also looks as if they wanted to get rid of the embarrassment of having him so near to home, even if it meant putting himself in the way of the enemies who were out to kill him. Then the gospel writer comments succinctly, *"Really his brothers had no confidence in him."* (7:5)

We must not jump to the conclusion from all this that the family of Jesus were not religious or interested in spiritual things. The reverse is more likely the case. Jesus had been brought up with a very thorough grounding in the Jewish faith. He knew the scriptures better than his contemporaries and he knew all the arguments, for and against, with respect to the most burning moral issues. But he had moved on by means of a unique personal relationship with God, by deep thought and reflection. He said things in his teaching that the folks at home could not understand, perhaps because they were too religious. They knew what their religion expected of them. They kept the Saturday Rest Day and the other festivals. They knew how to walk carefully to avoid breaking one of the multitude of the rules the Strict Set insisted on. Jesus, it seemed, did not care too much about all that. He even broke the rules of the Rest Day. He had been taught at home, no doubt, to avoid certain types of people, since 'sin' was contagious. But now he mixed with the very worst sort. He seemed to make a religion out of being kind to people. Weird!

The family of Jesus, or at least some of them, continued their custom of being in Jerusalem for the Passover. Maybe they stayed in one of the hotels, or in one of the villages outside Jerusalem that put up guests, possibly with relations or even camping out. We are told that Mary, his mother, was present at his execution, though she left before Jesus died and was taken down from the cross. It is not recorded that she visited the tomb. (Pictures of the mother of Jesus with her dead son in her arms are a pious invention, though they may be understood as spiritually or emotionally true. It was Maggie (Mary Magdala) who had Jesus in her arms. It was she, with Jo and Nick, who attended to his burial.)

Mary the mother of Jesus was entrusted to the care of his

special friend Larry who took her straightaway to his home. (It makes more sense that the beloved disciple was Lazarus rather than John the fisherman, for Lazarus lived with his two sisters, Mary and Martha at Dategrove (Bethany) just outside Jerusalem, whereas John's home was up in Galilee, a three day's walk. We know that John and the other Galilean disciples remained in Jerusalem for the next few days, at least.)

Has it ever struck you what a strange affair that was- Jesus entrusting his mother to his best friend? Presumably Mary would not have been in Jerusalem on her own. Some of her family would have been with her. More likely than not James, now her eldest son, would have accompanied her and made all the arrangements for the keeping of the Passover meal which was very much a family festival. What did James think about it when he learnt that his mother had been taken home by a complete stranger, instead of being restored to the bosom of her family? It wouldn't have been long before James arrived, possibly in a bad mood. His first words might have been, "What's going on then? What do you mean by abducting my mother?" His mother, albeit distraught, was an adult. There is no suggestion that she objected to Larry gently leading her away. This seems to have been planned by Jesus. Does it say something about Jesus' appraisal of his brother James? Did Jesus regard James as perhaps not the most suitable at dealing with their mother at her time of bereavement? Godly he may have been, but was he prone to be insensitive? Would he have quoted great chunks of scripture at his mother with lots of set prayers, interspersed by uncomplimentary comments about the one whose loss they both mourned, but neither completely understood? Since we know that Jesus always knew what he was doing, the odds are that he knew what he was doing on this occasion. He knew that from Larry and his sisters Mary and Martha, his Mum would get the very best in the way of befriending and bereavement counseling.

It is from Paul that we learn of the next significant event in the life of Jesus' brother. Paul was writing one of his letters to the Christian community in Corinth, Greece. He tells the Corinthian Christians that Jesus has returned to life from the dead. There is no doubt about the fact. Paul lists the people who had met with Jesus since the event, including Rocky and the other members of Jesus' inner circle of friends. Jesus was then seen on one occasion by over five hundred followers at once. After that, Jesus visited his brother James. Finally Paul met Jesus on the Damascus Road. It should be noted that James was not among the first batch of witnesses to the Resurrection. He was last but one named to Paul himself. Paul regarded himself as a latecomer to the experience. He described his meeting with Jesus as like to a difficult birth. *"Last of all, as to one untimely born, he appeared also to me"*. (1Corinthains 15:7 NRSV)

"He also visited his brother James, and all his close friends. Then, last of all, he came to me, though I didn't make things easy for him!" (Good As New).

Perhaps the meeting between Jesus and his brother James was difficult and dramatic as was the meeting between Jesus and the (then) Saul of Tarsus. But whereas the story of Paul's traumatic encounter on the Damascus Road was repeated often (by Paul and Luke), we are not given a shred of evidence, not the smallest hint, of what it was like between Jesus and James. Notice Paul only mentions James of Jesus' family. Neither Mary the mother, nor any one of Jesus' other brothers and sisters, are mentioned in the lists. Perhaps the appearance to James had to make do for the rest of them. He passed the news on. This suggests that there was something of a closeness between Jesus and James after all. Sometimes the closeness between two people is not recognized until one of them passes. The meeting of Jesus with James must have been a very private encounter. Nothing seems to have got out. It suggests, however, that despite past disagreements and misunderstandings, Jesus had some regard for his brother next-in-line. This understanding of the situation finds expression in 'The Gospel of Thomas' (Good As New 'Thought Provoking Sayings of Jesus" page 67.)

The friends of Jesus said to him, "We know you are going to leave us. What shall we do for a leader? Jesus said, "If you have any problems, you can always go to my brother James for advice. He's honest and fair. I think the world of him!"

This is important, probably early evidence of the respect James gained for himself in at least one of the first Christian communities. It seems like James reminded some of Jesus himself, and not only in looks. James was not involved, as far as we can tell, in the Day of Pentecost or the very first days of the Christian Church. But by the time Paul comes on the scene, is converted and becomes a missionary, James, Jesus' brother, has become the accepted leader of the church in Jerusalem. The church had been going through a crisis. There had been persecution that sent Christians, including their leaders, scattering in all directions. The experiment of living together communally had led to expenditure exceeding income, and the Jerusalem Christians were very poor. There were divisions. Steven had been martyred for radically suggesting the Jewish Law and Temple should be abolished. Others were very attached to the old ways and believed that being a Christian and being a good Jew were the same thing. It needed a firm hand, somebody with a bit of authority now the apostles had gone, to hold the church together. James, (unlike the other James – Jim, John's brother, of the 'Thunder and Lightning' duo) does not seem to have been a target for persecution at this time. That was almost certainly because he did nothing to offend his own people as Steven had done. I think we can safely call him a conservative.

James met Paul on several occasions. He was one of the first to recognize Paul's conversion and to back Paul's mission. However they were on opposite sides of the debate about how Jewish or non-Jewish Christianity should be. Paul's mission was to the Gentiles. He came to the conclusion that the Jewish Law was irrelevant to them. Indeed he believed that anyone, whether Jew or Gentile, who thought they could earn God's favor by keeping rules was mistaken. It was a simple trust in God's loving action in Jesus that brought a person into a relationship with God. Paul expressed these views in his letters. James too wrote a letter, probably for general distribution, in which he argued that 'faith without works is dead'. Paul's simple trust in Jesus was all very well, but that did not feed the hungry or clothe the naked. Some commentators think Paul and James were having a ding-dong in their letters. It is better to see that they just emphasize different aspects of the gospel- Paul, its basis in trust; James, its expression in deeds of kindness.

The question of how Jewish a Christian should be came to the crunch in a council held at Jerusalem. The main point at issue was whether the increasing number of new Gentile Christians should be obliged to keep the Jewish rules, particularly the one about cutting off the foreskin. The main leaders, Rocky, Paul, Cheery (Barnabas) and James skillfully held their fire, while those on both sides of the argument went for one another. Then Rocky got up and explained how the Spirit had inspired him to accept the first Gentiles on the same footing as the Jewish people. (Actually before Rocky was Philip the deacon who converted the Ethiopian, and before that, of course, Jesus himself.) Paul and Cheery were next to speak, giving an account of their successful missions among the Gentiles. Then we are told that James gave a summing up from the chair. James was speaking from the conservative side, whereas Paul and Cheery spoke from the liberal/radical side, and Rocky represented the charismatic 'follow the Spirit' approach, which, as Paul once reminded him, involved a typical 'rocky' approach, eating with Gentiles one minute and refusing to do so the next. (Letter to some Celtic Christians/Galatians 2:11) A split at this point in the Church's history could have resulted in three denominations or more.

The line James took was compromise. He understood the Jewish attachment to the law - he shared it. He also could see how it stood as a barrier to peoples of other cultures coming to God. He proposed that the Gentiles be asked to keep a few very basic rules. They should behave responsibly in the matter of sexual relations (the Gentiles were considerably more relaxed about sex than the Jewish people) and they should stick to kosher meat. There would be no obligation to be circumcised. James' final words are delightful. *"Moses doesn't need any more supporters. His words are read every Saturday in all our places of worship."* It's as if he's saying, "It's Jesus who needs supporters now!"

James probably saved the Church at that time. Because he had the trust and confidence of those who were attached to the old ways, he was able gently to lead them forward to a meeting point with those who were advocating new ways. He was the first great ecumenical- putting into practice his brother's prayer, "I pray that they may be ONE". Those who take the line, "No compromise", "No surrender", when it comes to ecumenical negotiations should be directed to the example of James. The Christian Church would never have survived without compromise. No one, just no-one, has all the truth!

However, we should add the proviso, 'As long as the compromise is not written on tablets of stone.' Then the compromise becomes another unbending truth, with its adherents 'orthodox' and its deviants 'heretics'. The very acceptance of compromise in the first place should mean an acceptance that what is agreed upon is provisional. The very fact that the first Christians agreed to accept Gentiles without their becoming Jews meant that the Jewish laws had already become provisional in Christian eyes. (Paul taught that the Law had been abolished – 'nailed by Christ to the cross'. Quaketown/Colossians 2:14. *'Jesus has scrapped the rules. He gave them a public execution.')* The Gentiles could not have been accepted without provisionality. The agreement at Jerusalem made a holding together possible for the time being. But later some disciples of Jesus would recall that Jesus had said it was not what entered a person that defiled them, but what came out. Mark says, 'These words of Jesus abolished the food laws at a stroke.' (7:14) This puts a different reflection on the Jerusalem compromise. It was not a compromise to allow the Gentiles to come in, but rather a compromise to keep sticky Old Testament Christians on board. It was they who were out of step with the teaching of Jesus, not Rocky or Paul. In fact the strictest of the Jewish Christians were probably lost, voting afterwards with their feet. And it cannot have been long before the Gentiles went all the way with Jesus and stopped being fussy about their food. Thanks (or otherwise) to Paul, the Gentile appreciation of sex as a leisure activity did receive a knock-out blow from which it is only just recovering, inflicting the churches with a big hangover headache. Compromise saved the day at Jerusalem and kept the middle together. That is all compromise can do. It is an essential Christian exercise, but only if it is regarded as a staging post and not a destination. As said Ron Davies, Secretary of State for Wales at the time when Wales voted by a whisker for a measure of devolution, "Devolution is not an event but a process." He was right. Devolution continues.

I was talking recently to an ecumenical enthusiast involved in meetings and discussions at the European level. There is a problem of coming to agreements with the eastern churches, since their outlook and ethos is so very different from that of the western churches, though, in their own way, they are very committed to the idea of Christian unity. My friend was telling me that the western churches had accepted into agreed documents, statements they did not believe to be true. If that is the case they are making a mistake. That is not a compromise but a concealment of the truth. The Church has frequently adopted that line and we are now suffering the consequences. Some Christians are waking up to the horrible realization that we have been telling the world lies for centuries. The trouble is that the world has realized first. Another problem is that many Christians could not care less. Christian unity has to be based on an awareness and acceptance of what each one of our divided companies genuinely believes to be true. If we continue to deal in lies and half truths we are lost. In the case where there are two irreconcilables, the two conflicting understandings of the truth should be set side by side, and we should await the verdicts of history and the Holy Spirit. A few years ago my present local church entered a new unity as a Baptist/United Reformed/Presbyterian 'uniting' church. There was a problem at the inauguration, since two out of the three denominations insisted that their statements of faith (somewhat lengthy) be read out publicly on that occasion. The members of the steering committee, to their dismay, found that the statements of faith were irreconcilable. Only the 'Vicar of Bray' could assent to them all. One said that Jesus Christ was the 'Supreme Authority', another said the Supreme Authority was 'The Word of God' which the wording made clear, was the Bible, both Old and New Testaments! Reconcile those two if you can. Our answer was for representatives of the three participating denominations to bring a copy each of their own statement and to lay it on the Communion Table in silence. They could think of no other way out. In my own mind and also in the mind of others, as we discussed it afterwards, it symbolized the Law once again being taken to the cross and nailed there with Christ. I refrain from saying what I think of those who drew the statements up in the first place.

Alas, the last piece of scriptural evidence relating to the career of James is less happy. Paul had come to Jerusalem to bring the money he had been collecting from the Gentile churches for the church in Jerusalem. James met him warmly, but he and others were anxious about the reception Paul would get from the hard-liners. They suggested that Paul make a gesture to please them. Although they recognized Paul's position on the Jewish Law - Paul counted it all as 'dung' in order to know Christ- a little compromise they felt was in order. If he were to attend the temple and be seen to take part in just one little Jewish ceremony, or back up a few brothers involved in it, it would go down very well with his critics. It was a bit like the advice given to Tony Blair to make a speech to the Women's Institute. (Best forgotten – it was a disaster!) Paul, because one of his principles was "All things to all people" and because he owed James a favor, agreed to do it. The plan did not work. Paul was set upon, a riot ensued, he was arrested and lost his freedom for the rest of his life. It was the first step on the road to trial at Rome and execution.

Why was it right for James to compromise on one occasion and wrong for Paul on another? Because the compromise James made was in the direction of the freedom and liberation Jesus came to bring, whereas the compromise Paul agreed to was in the direction of the bondage Jesus came to destroy. There is never any pleasing the old guard. Even James could not do it.

Fundamentalism is a blight on all religions. It always believes itself to be right, no compromise is possible. There are many kinds of fundamentalism, even within Christianity. Though they differ and vary among themselves, they all believe themselves to be in possession of absolute truth. There is Catholic fundamentalism, Protestant Evangelical fundamentalism and the fundamentalism of the fringe sects. It's wherever any basis, however apparently orthodox or Biblical, is adopted as immoveable and stands in place of and is more important than the love of God shown in Jesus. What happens if you try to compromise with a fundamentalist? You make a move to meet them, they step back so that you will have to move further, until they get you to that point where you surrender your freedom for their bondage. Though generally they would prefer you not to try to reach a rapprochement with them. Psychologically they are desperate to be the only ones who are right. That will not work if you agree with them. Fundamentalism is dangerous. All the churches have been hopelessly naive about it. I have watched the churches in my own denomination taken over one by one in my short time as a minister, 40 years. We have very few liberal churches left and probably fewer liberal ministers. Baptists were born in freedom, it is our most precious possession, the gift we should be bringing as our contribution to the whole Church, and we have all but lost it. And I would say to other churches where fundamentalists are regarded as an irritant or an amusing minority- It was so in my own denomination forty years ago. So watch it. They creep in, all smiles, all enthusiasm. They will identify those who they can get on their side by means of acts of kindness, just as they will identify those who are more of a challenge. They know how to make life uncomfortable for those who are 'unsound', and how to make it appear that it is others who are being uncharitable. They have an agenda; they know where they're going; they do not often fail. (I'm not making this up. Read the letters of Paul and you will find that's exactly how he experienced things. He felt himself persecuted by the 'worthier than thou' brigade, and he was!)

Poor James, he meant well. He tried to please his right wing, people with whom he felt some affinity. Instead his bright idea led to the arrest, imprisonment and death of a dear colleague. I bet he found it hard to forgive himself. God the Holy Spirit does have ways of getting around fundamentalists, so let's not be too downhearted. Paul's imprisonment gave him the leisure to write his letters in which the message of Christian freedom from the bondage of the law was preserved and handed on to future generations. Theologians thrown out by the Vatican, Christian writers banned from 'Christian' bookshops, may well turn out to be the prophets treasured by future generations. But there is no room for complacency. The Spirit calls us to be true to the Good News and to ensure that it is good news and not bad news. We have continually to seek the guidance of that same Spirit, to know when to compromise and when to avoid a trap.

You are the Vision

(1) You are the vision of what I could be,
Companion and Leader,- your love sets me free:
I hold you the first and the last in my heart;
Life will be gloomy if ever we part.

(2) If I need counsel, to you I must go;
When you walk beside me, the best paths you show;
Much closer than brother, more loyal than friend,
Travelling together, right on to the end.

(3) Rid me of weapons and angry displays;
Just help me rely on your methods always:
I need no defense but the truth and the light,
No strength or force but your love shining bright.

(4) Status means nothing, nor wealth or acclaim;
You only my meaning, my value, my fame;
Your care and compassion, your freedom from rules-
These, and these only, I need as my tools.

(5) Jesus, great-hearted, all-glorious in love,
Your gentleness puts you all others above;
I aim to be like you and let you control;
You are my vision: your New World my goal.

(After 'Be thou my vision' – Irish 8th century. Tune: Slane. Set to these words the last syllable of the 3rd line of each verse is slurred)

Chapter Twelve

"I told you so!"

At last the order came for us to sail to Italy. Julius, an officer in the Emperor's own troop, was put in charge of Paul and some other prisoners. We caught a boat making for the Asian ports on the Aegean sea, and set out straightaway. Paul had me and Harry from Tessatown for company. Next day, we landed at Sidon, and Julius kindly allowed Paul to go ashore to visit his Christian friends. They gave him some things he needed for the journey. We left Sidon and went east and north of Cyprus to avoid the full strength of the wind. Then we went along the mainland coast to the port of Myra. The officer found a boat on its way from Egypt to Italy and put us on board. The going was slow for the next few days, because we now had the full strength of the wind coming at us. We managed to get to Crete and struggled along the coast as far as a place called Fairhaven.

We were now very behind time and it was the middle of October, long past the season when it was safe to put to sea. Paul made his feelings known to those in charge. "Boys, it's too dangerous to go any further. We'll be putting the cargo and our lives at risk." But the officer was more inclined to listen to the boat-owner and the captain than to Paul. Most on board thought since Fairhaven was not a very good harbor to spend the winter in, it would be better to try to get to the port of Phoenix, further round the coast, which had a harbor protected from all winds. With a light wind behind them, they thought they would be able to make it. So they pulled up the anchor and started to work along the coast of Crete, keeping close to the shore. But suddenly a very strong wind, known locally as a 'north-eastern', came at us from the island. The boat could not turn into the wind, so we had to give way and be driven along. We used the small island of Gavdos to shield us from the full blast. Even so we got blisters on our hands, hauling in the dinghy. The next job was to send ropes underneath the boat to hold it together. The crew were afraid of being blown towards the sandbanks of north Africa, so they lowered all the rigging and allowed the boat to drift. Next day we made such heavy weather, the sailors started to throw the cargo overboard. On day three it was the turn of the boat's fittings to go over. It was too dark to see the sun or the stars for many days, and the storm showed no sign of slacking off. We thought we were done for!

It was a long time since anyone had had anything to eat. So Paul called for everyone's attention. "There you are, boys, - what did I tell you? If we'd stayed in Crete we wouldn't have got into this mess! My advice now is for you to keep your spirits up. We're going to lose the boat, but we're all going to stay alive. I had a message last night from the God who employs me and who I work hard for.'Don't lose your nerve, Paul, You're going to face the emperor. Those travelling with you will survive as well.' So cheer up, boys. I know God can be trusted to make it all come right. I expect we'll be castaways on an island somewhere."

We had been drifting for a fortnight and were somewhere in the Adriatic Sea. In the middle of the night the sailors had a hunch we were near to land. So they started to measure the depth of the water with a weight and line. They found it was quite shallow, and a further testing showed even shallower. They were afraid the boat might end up on the rocks, so they let down four anchors from the back of the boat, and hoped they would live to see another day. Then the sailors tried to play a dirty trick. They lowered the dinghy saying they were going to put down the anchors from the front of the ship. But really they meant to escape. Paul shouted to the soldiers with their officer, "If the sailors don't stay on board, there'll be no chance of surviving!" So the soldiers cut the ropes of the dinghy and it drifted away. It was nearly day and Paul tried to get everybody to have something to eat. He said, "You've been in a state of tension for a fortnight without eating anything. You need to eat something to build up your strength. You're all going to escape without a scratch." Then Paul took a piece of bread and held it up for all to see. He said 'thank you' to God, broke the bread and started eating. This *boosted morale, and everybody on board joined in, two hundred and seventy-six in all. When they had eaten all they wanted, they threw the cargo of wheat into the sea to make the boat lighter.*

When it was light, nobody recognized the coast, but they saw a sandy cove and thought it might be possible to get the boat to run aground there. They cut off the anchors and left them in the sea, and got the oars ready. Then they put up the sail in front of the boat and we started to move towards the beach. But we got stuck on some rocks under the water. The front of the boat would not move, but the back was being broken by the waves. The soldiers wanted to kill the prisoners to stop them swimming away. But the officer would not let them, because he wanted to save Paul. He ordered all those who could swim to jump overboard and swim to land. The rest followed using planks and rafts made from pieces of the boat. That's how we all managed to get ashore safely.2Luke chapter 27.

When we read the accounts of the times Luke was the traveling companion of Paul, when Luke uses 'we' instead of 'they', the impression we get is that Luke loved Paul very much and admired his abilities and zeal. At the same time, we can tell that sometimes Paul irritated Luke greatly. People we love often have that effect on us. Somehow their failings are more difficult to accept than the failings of those who do not mean much to us.

Luke tells the story of a shipwreck from which he and Paul were survivors. Luke expands his narrative to relate in full the details of the weather, the course of the ship and the desperate efforts of the sailors and soldiers to get the ship under control and to prevent loss of life. The two friends, Luke and Paul, were not just spectators. They joined with the crew in handling the ropes. The Greek text suggests they worked so hard that they rubbed the skin off their hands. Paul, true to form, did not confine his assistance to tugging at the ropes. He had advice to offer. This is where we sense that Luke found Paul difficult to cope with as a friend. We hear him saying, underneath his breath, "Shut up, Paul! Leave it to those who know what they are doing!" Luke does not admit to saying this out loud, of course. He may have done, or perhaps he thought it wiser to hold his tongue.

Paul liked giving advice and he believed his special position as a helper of Jesus gave him the right to express his opinion, even on practical matters that had nothing to do with theology. Paul had been to sea many times before, so he thought this gave him the necessary experience to advise the captain. He had a point. They found themselves facing disaster at sea because Paul's previous advice had been ignored. After they had been delayed by bad weather and obliged to take shelter in Crete, Paul had told the captain it was unwise to continue the voyage to Rome so late in the year. But the captain had been deaf to Paul's pleading. Paul relished his opportunity to say, "I told you so!"

"There you are, boys – what did I tell you? If we'd stayed in Crete we wouldn't have got into this mess!"

Luke blushes and carries on with his job of swabbing the excess water from the deck, or whatever. We all enjoy the opportunity to say 'I told you so!'. It is never a good thing to do. It is bad psychology. People will forgive us many times for being wrong. It is harder to forgive someone for being right. The captain and his crew remembered well enough what Paul's advice had been, without him rubbing it in. Self-righteousness takes many forms, and being wiser than others before the event is one of them. There are many politicians, as well as ordinary members of the public, who could see quite well the sort of mess the governments of USA and the UK would get into in Iraq if they embarked on an invasion of that country, especially without the help and backing of the United Nations. Those politicians who were wiser than their fellows get little credit for their wisdom, and if they wish to preserve their reputation for wisdom, they must not harp on and on about what it is now too late to do anything about. They do not even have the consolation that future leaders will learn from the mistake. The only lesson we learn from history is that the leaders of nations never learn the lessons of history. Alas, every generation has to make its own mistakes, and they are usually the same mistakes as last time round. Violence *always* leads to violence. There has never been any exception. 'When will they ever learn?'

Beware, parents, if you are anxious about your wayward young adults. Sometimes wisdom means holding your tongue and a neutral expression. Beware, if, like me in times past, you look after people whose behavior is constantly getting them into trouble. They are only too aware of what they have just done wrong. There's no need to tell them!

Luke is a brilliant writer. But we miss much of his subtlety unless we read between the lines. It is also important to keep looking back over what he has already written. You cannot understand Luke's thoughts and feelings in chapter 27, unless you go back and have a good read of chapter 21. Paul, like Ollie of 'Laurel and Hardy', vents his frustration by saying, "Here's another right mess you've got me into."But the messes the comic duo got into were the results of their joint efforts, as fans of their pictures will know. So too there is rarely one person who can be regarded as responsible for a crime, or indeed a life of crime. J.B. Priestly's play 'An Inspector Calls' teaches us that life is much more complicated than that. Those who blame their backgrounds, the ill treatment they received from parents, unfair economic and educational systems, and so on, are, of course, wishing to dodge their own responsibility. But they are on very strong ground. The individual prisoner is a scapegoat, consciously or unconsciously aware of it. Each prisoner does time for a multitude of people who share responsibility for the prisoners' crime, as will be revealed if the Last Judgment turns out according to the pattern traditionalists anticipate. Such would indeed be a scary event. No one would escape, except perhaps those who have received more than their fair share of punishment in this life. Jesus must have understood this when he said, 'The first shall be last and the last shall be first'. The message of scripture is also that in some, incomprehensible way, the firm of God and Jesus lifts the responsibility from off our shoulders. I stress 'incomprehensible' since I do wish theologians would not keep trying to explain it, often in the crudest and most inadequate of theological language.

> *'Tis mystery all, let earth adore*
> *And angel minds inquire no more!'*
> (Charles Wesley)

Why did Paul and his companions suffer shipwreck on this particular occasion? Who was responsible? Why were they on this journey to Rome in the first place? It's a long story. But Luke gives us an idea where it all started in chapter 21. If there is any chapter in which Luke boldly criticizes his friend and mentor Paul, this is it.

Paul was determined to go to Jerusalem. He had some money to deliver to the Jerusalem Christians, a gift he had collected from the churches overseas. Was this God's will? Luke makes it very clear that, no, it was not God's will. Luke describes how he and Paul dropped off at Tyre on the way. He says,

*We found out where the Christians were living, and stayed with them for a week. They gave Paul a message from the Spirit. **She said Paul should not go to Jerusalem.** After our stay in Tyre, we got ready to continue our journey.*(Verses 4&5)

There are no two ways about it. Luke states in no uncertain terms, that Paul gets clear advice from God's Spirit that he must not go to Jerusalem. Paul defies the Spirit's advice and persists on his own course. Paul receives an instruction from the highest quarter and deliberately disobeys. Later, continuing their travel by boat, Paul and company get off at Caesartown and stay with Philip- not the apostle, but the one skilled in spreading the 'Good News', and also, you will recall, skilled in watching out for and obeying God's leading. Philip had four daughters who were also gifted at receiving and handing on messages from God. They were visited by Hopper (his Greek name 'agabus' means 'locust'). Hopper was an honored 'prophet', the very prophet who had predicted the famine that had led to Paul's decision to make a collection for the Jerusalem Christians in the first place. Paul was thus in the company of specialists in knowing and interpreting the mind of God through the Spirit. Hopper knew what a stubborn customer Paul could be. So he did not confine himself to words. He used the method of the Hebrew prophets, especially Isaiah and Jeremiah. He made a dramatic, physical gesture. He snatched off Paul's belt and tied Paul's hands and feet with it. Then he said,

"I've got this message from God's Spirit. She says, 'This is how the people of Jerusalem will tie up the one this belt belongs to and take him as a prisoner to the Romans.' " (verse 11)

Luke goes on, *'When we heard this we all tried to argue Paul out of going to Jerusalem.'* This makes it clear that Luke's sense of the Spirit was at one with that of Hopper, as was that of Philip and his four Spirit attuned daughters. Paul's reply gives us some clue as to why he persisted in ignoring advice from God's Spirit.

"All this crying is breaking my heart. I'm quite willing to become a prisoner and even to die in Jerusalem if it helps the cause of Jesus, my Leader."

So that's what Paul was up to. He wanted to do a Jesus! Jesus had boldly set his face towards Jerusalem, - so would Paul!

I recall a seminar I was privileged to be a part of amongst the students of Westcott House, Cambridge, on a visit there way back in the 1970s. The subject for discussion among the ordinands was,

"How can we be Christ to our people?" I think I made some protest as a Protestant Nonconformist. I did not think it was the calling of a member of the clergy to be Christ. I still do not think so. Jesus will sometimes be incarnate in the stranger, in the child, in the persecuted, in the oppressed, but in each case the person themselves will not be aware of it. Neither will anyone else at the time. To think you can be Jesus, or even stand in for Jesus, means you have to be lacking in humility, and that in itself will bar you from the exercise. Paul on this occasion was in a headstrong, arrogant mood. He would not listen to his fellow Christians. *"All this crying is breaking my heart..!!!* It was a pity Paul would not allow the tears of his friends to break his stubborn self-will.

Paul went to Jerusalem. But he did not behave like Jesus. Luke, by means of his researches for his Gospel, part one, knew how Jesus behaved. Jesus kept silent in court. He refused to defend himself before the High Priest, Pilate or Herod. He submitted to the cross. The moment Paul was arrested he used it as a publicity exercise to get his views to the Jewish leaders, and then when there was a danger of his being convicted or torn apart limb from limb by the mob, he used his special privilege as a Roman citizen to get his case transferred to Rome. The Caesar Paul thought he was appealing to was Claudius, the best of the appalling Julian-Claudian House. Claudius had a reputation for being a conscientious and fair judge. Paul was not to know that by the time he got to Rome, or soon after, Claudius would be succeeded by his nephew Nero! Paul wrote chapter 13 of Romans with Claudius in mind. It is difficult to imagine him saying 'The Powers that be are ordained of God' if Nero or Caligula had been on the throne. Anyhow, as Luke skillfully shows us, Paul ended up being shipwrecked. Luke and the other invaluable members of the mission team, as well as Paul himself, were at risk of a watery grave, because Paul disobeyed the advice of God's Spirit. As Luke describes Paul blaming captain and crew for not taking his wise advice, he condemns himself. Had Paul taken the advice given to him in the name of the Spirit by Luke, among others, they would not have been on this particular ship in the first place. No wonder Luke was muttering underneath his breath. We can imagine how he felt! But let us not lose sight of the more important point, more important than the matter of making mistakes or owning up to them. None of us is up to being Jesus. We can do our best to copy him in some respect or other. Do what he did, we cannot. Not even Paul was up to it.

Jesus described God for us as a parent or friend. Since the performance of human parents and friends is variable, it is important to add that Jesus intends us to understand that God is better than the best parent or friend our minds or experience can imagine. Human parents do not reach the heights of God's parenting. They do not naturally behave like the father in Jesus' story of the adventurous son; though some parents who know the story may do their best to copy God's parenting in their dealings with their children. Thus we must quash the bad press, given by some who enthusiastically claim to represent God, which describes God as poised to inflict a selection of unpleasant events on us, the moment we step out of line. The best parents and friends are not like that, only the worst. God loves us and cares for us in the context of a mutual relationship. If we act as if God's loving care for us does not exist, as Paul did when he ignored the loving advice of his friends, we may well have a shipwreck or two, and it is not sporting of us to try to shift the blame like Paul. But all is not lost, however we react. God picks up on the relationship and shows us how to make the best of things from that point on. It's as if God has a plan 'A', a plan 'B' and a plan 'C' etc. etc., just in case.

In the story Luke relates, a string of unfortunate events, for which more than one person shares the responsibility, leads to the moment where Paul, Luke and a ship full of people are shortly to go on the rocks. In this situation, once he's got the hypocritical "I told you so" off his chest, Paul is superb. When everybody else is panicking and giving up all hope, he takes charge, addressing the company calmly and firmly. He stops the foolish attempt of a group to make a dash for it on their own in the lifeboats. Then he tells the passengers and crew that the best thing they can do in view of the fact that they are going to need all their energies, is to have something to eat. It seems they had not eaten properly for a fortnight. No one was hungry. Fear and panic do not go with a healthy appetite. Now it is Paul's turn to beg. Now it is his turn to urge and plead in tones of love and concern, as his friends at Caesartown had previously done when they had his best interests at heart. No one made a move towards the table on which Paul had put some bread. So Paul began the meal himself. The words Luke uses to describe what was happening are familiar.

Then Paul took a piece of bread and held it up for all to see. He said 'thank you' to God, broke the bread and started eating.

Luke is recounting a Communion Service aboard ship. Do we locate here the origin of the 'Sursum Corda' ('Lift up your hearts'), which is frequently used at services of Holy Communion? For we are told, that Paul's action *'boosted morale'.* The assembled company 'took heart'. There follows a fully inclusive communion, after the mind and intention of Jesus. *'And everybody on board joined in, two hundred and seventy-six in all,'* sharing the bread that Paul had blessed and broken – sailors, soldiers, passengers, the other prisoners, merchants, galley slaves, Gentiles, God fearers, Pagans, Atheists – the lot. Incidentally, in addition to the origin of the Sursum Corda, we may also have here the origin of the practice of the officiant being the first to take the communion. Unfortunately, it would seem that an act of encouragement and example from Paul has been turned by the Church into an act of priestly privilege and bad table manners.

This account of a very unusual communion, in very extreme

and frightening conditions, abounds in Eucharistic touches, including registering the numbers communicating, which some churches still do. The numbers were counted at the communions with the five thousand and the four thousand, both figures being rounded up in order to give them special significance. On Paul's ship the numbers were 276, which we are probably to understand, like all the numbers in the gospels, to be symbolic. Like the 153 fish caught on the morning Jesus conducted communion on the shore of the lake in Galilee, the number is triangular. You can make an equilateral triangle out of the numbers, beginning with 1,2,3…etc as from the top to the bottom of a pyramid. A triangle is a symbol suggesting 'not-yet-complete'. It is on the way to a square, the symbol of completeness. The mission of the Christian community is in full swing. There is room for more, even on a boat about to sink, because those on board do not ultimately depend on anything material for their safety, but on the one who has said 'I will never leave you or forsake you'. Sometimes the boat has to sink or flounder on the rocks for God's people to realize that it is on Jesus they depend and not on an organization. Whereas, at the feeding of the crowds of day-trippers in the desert, there was care to pick up discarded scraps – a message for our current careless and wasteful civilization, - after the communion on board ship, when everyone has had sufficient, the surplus is thrown overboard to lighten the ship. There is a time for careful preserving of our provisions 'waste not, want not', as we oldies were taught in wartime. But there are times when the Church finds itself encumbered by excess baggage. Then we must have the courage to throw overboard what we do not need. Our church buildings are today like so many worn out outdated battleships, expensive, beyond refurbishment and unsuited to our require-ments. The Church is struggling for its life, and its life has to do with people not rigging, or bricks and mortar. We are living in architecturally impressive slums. Most of the ships in our ecclesi-astical fleet need to go the way of the Royal Yacht Britannia.

Together with the outmoded attitudes of Christians in the matter of human relationships, our attitude to the accommodation we have inherited is an immense handicap to the progress of God's New World. Add to that the baggage of so much of our incomprehensible and eccentric theology and liturgy, appreciated only by the dwindling numbers of spiritual 'anoraks' who just about keep our doors open, and boy, are we up against it! Despite all his faults, Paul was one of the best ever followers of the Leader who said (more than once probably), "Destroy this temple!" When Paul sensed that his ship was heading for the rocks, he first boosted the energy and morale of his fellow passengers, then prepared them to jump. One feels that Paul's response to the crisis he faced somewhere in the middle of the Mediterranean about two thousand years ago would do well as a sane and spiritual agenda for responsible leaders of the Church today.

Paul was superb in an emergency. By taking and eating the bread (a gesture both ritual and nerve-calming), then the invitation "Come and get it", all of which he believed he had received from Jesus himself, Paul presided over a strengthening and healing experience of Holy Communion. The communion service means nothing unless it stands as an invitation to everyone in sight to join in.

At the height of the troubles in what was still the Soviet Union, but not for much longer, when President Gorbachev had been taken prisoner and the tanks of the Communist reactionary forces were out in Red Square threatening the freedom demonstrators, some Russian Orthodox priests took the consecrated bread and wine on to the streets and offered it to the men in the tanks. The men were old-style Communists, almost certainly professed atheists, yet they were offered the bread and the wine. Whether it was this gesture that did the trick, defusing a terrifying situation, it is probably unwise to be dogmatic about it. But shortly after the men came out of the tanks and the crisis was over.

The line Paul and the Russian priests took in an emergency,

Christians should adopt as regular practice.Not, 'The things of God for the people of God', but 'The things of God for everybody'.
Another miracle on the waters:-

Twists the Tornado

Twists the tornado over the lake;
Efforts in vain, they're bound to sink;
As for the captain, he's asleep,
Still and calm.

"Wake up, all's lost", in terror cry
the seasoned sailors, set to die;
Jesus stands tall, his voice raised high,
"Hush, keep calm!"

The wild wind drops, the angry sky
lightens, and waves rock lullaby;
The sweating oarsmen heave a sigh
At the calm.

When panic tries to make us slip,
Threatening to sink our leaky ship,
Steady us in your mighty grip,
Source of calm.

(After Godfrey Thring. 1823-1903. Tune St. Aelred in C minor.
**Amend first four notes of melody to ascending arpeggio: middle
C, Eb, G, upper C.)**

Chapter Thirteen

Snake – Friend or Foe?

When we were all safely on dry land, we found we were on the island of Malta. The people there were very kind to us. It had started to rain and it was very cold, and they lit a fire and welcomed us all round it. Paul had twisted together a bundle of sticks to put on the fire. The heat frightened an adder out of the wood and it clung to Paul's wrist. When the local people saw the snake hanging from Paul's hand, they whispered together, "This man must be a murderer. He's escaped from the sea, but he's not going to escape justice." But Paul shook the snake into the fire. The snake had done him no harm. The people were expecting Paul to swell up any minute or fall down dead, but when, after a while, it was obvious nothing of the kind was going to happen, they altered their opinion of Paul and started calling him a god.

Near the place we came ashore were the estates of the ruler of Malta, who was called Lee. He invited us to his home and looked after us with great kindness for three days. At that time his father was suffering from gastric fever and had to stay in bed. Paul went to his room, put his arms round him, and asked God to make him better. As soon as he recovered, everyone else on the island who had an illness came to see Paul, and they were all made better. The islanders treated us like royalty, and when the time came to set out to sea again, they brought onto the boat everything we needed for the voyage.'28: 1-10.

For a few days one summer Valerie and I paid a visit to Ynys Môn (Anglesey), the large island in the North West corner of Wales. Part of Ynys Môn is in turn an island off the island, 'Holy Island', including the port of Caergybi (Holyhead). We were blessed with good weather, and one day climbed the Holyhead Mountain – the only mountain in Ynys Môn, from where we were able to get a marvelous view of the whole island spread before us. After the energy expended on the steep and rocky ascent, we came down to a cliff overlooking the bright blue sea. We took off our shoes, laid our coats on the short grass and went to sleep, just a little distance away from one another. In my sleep, I felt something soft on the inner side of my leg, and still asleep I said to myself, "That feels like a snake." I woke up to find a very large adder making its way up my legs and onto my tummy. I jumped up backwards and the adder dropped onto the grass in front of me. I shouted to Valerie who also jumped up. The adder made no attempt to move away. I was in a bit of a quandary, since I had removed my glasses and they were now lying close to the adder's head. Somehow I felt no fear…I bent down and retrieved my glasses. Still the adder made no movement – no hissing, no curling up into a striking position. Valerie got her camera and took a photograph, which we have since had enlarged and put on the wall on the landing. It is the record of what I felt then, and continue to feel, was a friendly visitation on the part of the snake. You can almost see a smile on her face, as if to say, "Don't be afraid, I only want to welcome you to my home." It was some while before the adder decided to slither away, very slowly over my jacket and into the long grass further away. (Later I confirmed the female sex of the adder from a nature book by her slightly darker, duller coloration. Incidentally, and mercifully irrelevant to the story, the poison from the bite of a female adder is stronger than that of a male!)

I had always been afraid of snakes. I shuddered as I watched those brave people on the telly in animal programs, wrapping great pythons around their necks. Somehow I have not been so afraid of snakes since that encounter with my friendly Holyhead snake. One of my piano pupils, a lad who is very fond of animals, including rats and reptiles, asked me if I would like to see his coral snake. I said, "Yes, I would, please." His parents were appalled. They did not share his love of God's slithery creatures. They winced as I stroked the snake and let him scent my hand with his tongue. But my pupil was impressed. It seems I was the only one of his friends or acquaintances who had reacted to his truly beautiful pet in this positive way.

Adders can give a very nasty bite, on occasions fatal. But they are not, according to the nature books, aggressive creatures. Fear of snakes is one of the most frequent of phobias and goes deep into our common human culture. The scriptures have not done anything to remove this fear. Evil appears in the form of a snake in the third chapter of Genesis, and Satan is referred to as 'that old snake' in the book of Revelation. Both John the Dipper and Jesus refer to the strict set (Pharisees) as a 'viper's nest', and the description is not meant to be complimentary. However, ability to handle snakes is one of the specialties of the Christian according to a made-up addition to Mark's version of the Good News. The writer may have had snakes of the human variety in mind, or in the case of biological snakes have been indicating the reconciliation of nature in Jesus, God's Chosen. Jesus lived for an extended period of time with the wild beasts in the desert without coming to any harm. The Hebrew prophet Isaiah foresaw a time when wolves and lambs would contentedly lie down together, and when "a baby will not be harmed if playing near a poisonous snake."

If you have a go at a snake with a stick then the snake will use what defenses nature has given it. But it is not the snake that represents evil, but that fear of the snake which leads to aggressive and irrational behavior on our part. The conquest of evil involves the conquest of fear and irrational prejudices. In the seventeenth century Christians burnt women alive for fear they were witches. These were sometimes women of high intelligence with special skills in the healing arts. Today some Christians with the same blind zeal persecute gay people. Blind, because they do not even realize they are persecuting. Often their attitude leads to the death or the mental collapse of one or more human beings, while they go blithely on, 'loving the sinner and hating the sin' as they put it. They are hosts to what is now recognized medically as an irrational phobia against, in many cases, the most gentle and sensitive representatives of humankind.

I have great sympathy with the Quaker, who in a debate in which we were urging one another to fight racism, perhaps by joining an organization such as 'Christians Against Racism', said she would rather not be considered as being *against* anything. She conceived of the Christian's role as being *for* that which is good. Her point is very important. The danger of seeing the Christian life as a fight against evil, as many Christians do, is that we can all too easily mistake the precise point at which evil is making itself manifest. It is not the snake that is evil, nor the snake's bite, but what causes the snake to bite. Jesus had a lot to say about bad behavior beginning in the 'heart'. Sexual exploitation does not begin in the abusive acts themselves, nor in the stirring of the sexual organs. It begins in those attitudes we inherit, or in which we are trained or adopt from our peers, which degrade others into something less than sons and daughters of God.

In Luke's second volume we have the story of a snake who did Paul no harm at all. Paul saw the snake not as one of God's creatures, beautifully and wonderfully made, but as a threat. In his first volume Luke records the words of Jesus about God's care for individual sparrows (12:16) as does the gospel of Matthew, with the added comment that God takes note of every sparrow that comes to grief – probably a criticism of their slaughter in the sacrificial system. (10: 29-31) Was Luke capable of applying these words in his mind to the care of God for an individual viper on the island of Malta? Paul, who tells us elsewhere to fight evil with good (Romans 12:21), destroyed the snake. The onlookers regarded it as a good act, and it may be that Luke regarded it as such too. But we should see it as a bad act and learn from it to identify and weed out our destructive instincts.

All things bright and beautiful

(Opening chorus)
All things bright and beautiful,
And those we count less worth,
Whether grey or colorful,
God loves the whole round earth.

(Chorus thereafter)
Whether dull or beautiful,
The outsize and the small,
Commonplace or wonderful,
God loves and cares for all.

1. The pine trees up in Scotland,
The palm trees down in Spain;
The sunflowers and the snowdrops,
The heat-waves and the rain.

2. The onions in the garden,
The potted plants we buy,
The rock pools by the seaside,
The white gulls floating high.

3. God loves the creepy crawlies
And things that bite and sting;
The spider with her lace work,
The snake with patterned skin.

4. The people who are moody,
And those brim full of fun;
The strong folk and the gentle,
God loves us every one.

5. Variety is God's purpose.
And difference is God's choice;
God made the soaring tenor
And deep contralto voice.

6. As well as eyes outside us,
We have some inside eyes,
So we can share God's vision
And mark each day's surprise.

(After 'All things bright and beautiful' C. F. Alexander 1818-95)

Chapter Fourteen

Books, Hair and Foreskin.

BOOKS

God helped Paul to do many remarkable things. When towels or cloths Paul had used were taken to people who were ill, they got better, and those who were confused were able to think clearly again.

A group of Jewish healers, who advertised themselves as the sons of one of the leading clergy in Jerusalem called Sheba, went around from place to place offering to cure people. Once they tried to help some mentally disturbed people by using the name of Jesus. They said, "We're going to put you right in the name of Jesus, the one Paul talks about." One of them shouted back, "I've heard of Jesus and Paul, but who are you?" Then the healers were attacked violently. They ran out of the house badly beaten and without their clothes.

When the people of Ephesus in both the Jewish and Greek communities got to hear about this, they were impressed, and the reputation of Jesus, the Leader, increased. Many who became Christians admitted to doing things they were ashamed of. Some of them had dabbled in black magic. They burned their books in front of everybody. These books were very valuable - enough to employ a thousand workers for a year. This shows the value that was now being put on the truth from God.(2Luke 19: 11- 20)

There is some doubt as to how and why the great library of ancient Alexandria came to be destroyed. According to one account, when in 642 the Arab general Amr took the city, he received a request from a Coptic priest, John the Grammarian, for the books. This led Amr to write to the Caliph Omar to ask what the fate of the books should be. The reply came, "About the books you mention, if what is written in them agrees with the Book of

God, they are not required; if it disagrees, they are not desired. So destroy them." Thereupon Amr ordered the books to be distributed among the baths of Alexandria to be used as fuel for heating. Recently historians have cast doubt on the authenticity of this story. It did not come to light until the twelfth century, the time of the crusades, and may have been a piece of propaganda used in the war of words between east and west. Prior to this it may have been propaganda on the part of one Islamic sect against another – Shi'ite against Sunni. (The Sunni Saladin sold famous libraries to pay his troops.) If the story is true, then it must be counted as an aberration since the Muslims are to be credited with great traditions of library building begun under the leadership of the Caliphs of Baghdad.

Whatever the history, and whoever was responsible for the tragic loss of the ancient world's greatest library, the words attributed to the Caliph Omar stand as a classic statement of religious fundamentalism, - extreme, but chillingly accurate. It does not matter whether the fundamentalism is Christian, Muslim, Hindu or Jewish, the concept of truth is the same. Truth is only to be found within a narrow body of truth revealed supernaturally, uncontaminated by human error, once and for all. Anything else claiming to be truth is irrelevant or a threat. It cannot be flirted with; it must be destroyed.

In Luke's second volume there is a story of books being burnt. It is part of a longer story of religious intolerance. The atmosphere is that of superstition and panic. Paul – or perhaps more accurately, Paul's campaign managers – were encountering the threat of competition. They were doing quite well with their cloths and towels taken from Paul (with his knowledge and permission, we wonder?) These objects were proving very effective folk remedies! However, a rival group of Jews were practicing healing on the same patch. No mention of cloths or towels. These were relying simply on the effectiveness of the name of Jesus. How unsound! Up to this point they must have had some success, but now they were presented with a case too hot to handle. Their humiliating failure was regarded by their cloth waving rivals as proof positive of their heresy. Whether or not Luke agrees with this verdict we cannot say. He was a qualified Greek doctor and probably had his reservations about both groups. But he creates a very vivid picture of a community in which reason and open mindedness have, for the time being at least, been jettisoned. In his first volume Luke records the incident in which the disciples asked Jesus to stop somebody from healing in his name because whoever he or she was did not belong to their team. Jesus replied, "That was wrong of you. You should have recognized someone like that as your ally." (9:49-50) This is part of the material Luke obtained from Mark and added to his first volume after he had completed his second volume. Did he give a wry smile as he recalled 'Sheba and Sons, Effective Cures Ltd?'

Once the cry of 'heresy' is raised there is a predictable chain reaction – fear, people falling over one another to admit their guilt, and the attempt to silence the adversary. In order to stamp out opposing ideas, there was, in Ephesus, a public burning of books. So began the 'Christian' tradition of censorship. However, Paul's name is not linked with the exercise and he does not appear to have been present. The fact that we are not told who was in charge suggests that none of the prominent leaders with names familiar to us, or to Luke for that matter, were present to exercise caution or restraint.

Books were much more precious in those days than they are now. If someone took the trouble to write or copy a book it was unlikely to be frivolous or for the purposes of sensationalism. It would be because the author or copyist believed there was something of great value to be conveyed. Books were scarce and highly prized because the standard was high. What these books of 'magic' contained we cannot know, but it is unlikely they were simply lists of quaint spells and mumbo-jumbo. The price of this haul was valued at fifty thousand times the average daily wage of a farm laborer. An Alexandria in miniature! These books almost certainly contained, amongst other things, some of the secrets of Greek medicine, unequalled until recent times, and they may well have contained aspects of science and mathematics which had they been studied and built upon might have prevented some of the darkness of the dark ages. Had Christianity been prepared to take on board and wrestle with what might have appeared at first to be threatening alternatives of the truth, then many future stupid blunders might have been avoided and the true fundamentals of the faith identified instead of being cluttered by incidentals.

Christians, and indeed Muslims, who may well have caught the bug from us, are still trying to defend the truth by trying to cut truth's vital air supply – freedom. The claims of Darwin cannot be debated in a calm reasonable manner – they must be ruled out of order before the debate starts. The Christian, instead of asking what truth can be learnt from Darwin, only asks how can Darwin be effectively put to the flames. This brings just contempt from those who have a respect for reason and induces all kinds of guilt and confusion amongst those who have both a Christian commitment and a commitment to science. It probably postpones the date when the weaknesses as well as the strengths of Darwin can be assessed, since the debate has been sidetracked into an irrelevancy. The same can be said of Freud and Marx whose weaknesses have been exposed but whose strengths have never been understood or appreciated by Christians in the main, to their great detriment. The attitude of many Christians to the researches of psychiatry and sociology is lamentable. So are the responses of Christians to much that is challenging and new in the realm of the arts. The response of Islam (not all Islam) to Salman Rushdie's *Satanic Verses*, found its parallel in the response of many Christians to Scorcese's film *The Last Temptation*. Blind anger in both cases made it impossible for the devotee to discern new angles on the truth and the exposing of naiveté that were being offered. More recently *The Jerry Springer Opera* was condemned largely because of the aversion of Christians to *'blasphemy'* and *'bad language'*, whereas the musical was in fact a satirical critique of the 'Jerry Springer Show' itself and raised important questions about 'Reality TV' and the chaotic state of personal relationships today. It also had many striking affinities with the Book of Job, which those who bash rather than read their Bibles failed to notice. The Harry Potter books and films are condemned because they contain magic, wizards and witches (so did Enid Blyton). Harry Potter is as much Christian allegory as C.S Lewis, as will one day be realized. Again, a lot stems from church-goers who do not know their Bibles, or even, it would seem, the basic plot of the gospels, and allow themselves to be intimidated by bullies who pretend they do. All this does not mean that Christians have to find some good or some message in everything that is proffered by science or culture, but it means we should not form an opinion until we have listened, reflected, listened and reflected again.

Heine, the German poet (1797-1856) said, "People who burn books end up burning people." Thus the burning of books in Acts 19 strikes us as unpleasantly foreboding. It would not be too long before the Church would be burning people who had stumbled on some truth the Church found uncomfortable. Books are burnt because they contain ideas. When the books are no more the ideas live on in the minds of people. So they are next in line. Jesus was well aware in his controversies with the religious people of his day that what he was facing was authoritative ignorance that he described on many occasions as darkness. The closed eyes, the refusal to see new truth when it is presented to view, produces a darkness of the mind that doubles in on itself. Luke was well aware of this frustration in the ministry of Jesus. He alone records a section of the encounter between Jesus and the Council in which Jesus expressed his weariness at the impossibility of having a meaningful debate with people who have already made up their minds.

In the morning there was a meeting of the councilors and clergy. They had Jesus brought before them. They said to him, "If you're God's Chosen, then tell us." Jesus said, "You've already formed your opinion, so what's the point in telling you anything? You're not open to a meeting of minds.(1Luke 22:66)

Luke also had his own version of the words of Jesus about the eyes being the lamp for the body.

"We see with our eyes. If you've got good eyesight, your whole body can move around freely. If you've got bad eyesight, you'll bump into things. So get your eyes checked! In other words, be honest with yourself. Then you'll have a light inside you shining outwards, like a lamp. Everything happening around you will be clear to you." (11:34)

This suggests that Luke, who was an intelligent, educated man, knew the processes whereby truth could be discovered or suppressed. He knew that truth could only come to someone with an open mind, and that it is the closed mind that crucifies. He must have been uneasy at the loss of all those books.

HAIR

After a long stay in Corinth, Paul said goodbye to his Christian friends in the town and went by sea to Syria. Cill and Will went with him. Paul had been letting his hair grow long to show he was on special duties for God. But at the seaport he had his hair cut short again before boarding the boat. When they arrived at Ephesus, Paul decided to put Will and Cill in charge of operations there and leave them to it. (2Luke 18: 18)

It was in Pontypridd, in 1969, when Baptists and Congregationalists had just merged to bring into being

'Pontypridd United Church' of which I had been inducted the minister. One of the deacons I acquired as a result of this bold, and, for our part of the world, novel venture, was an ex-schoolmistress, prominent to overpowering. She had done a good job for many years in a Secondary Modern school, a type of school designed for those who failed the 11+ exam and thus deemed to have proved themselves to be short of brains, but possibly capable of being trained to be skilled workers. I failed the 11+ and attended Secondary Modern schools for three years before being spotted as potential academic material and moved to the Grammar School. Thus I am an ardent supporter of Comprehensive education, but also hold at the same time that my sojourn in the Secondary Modern was God's way of teaching me to make friends with and relate to people who were not academic, and also, in many cases, underprivileged and despised. I made my way eventually to Oxford by way of Southampton managing to pick up two good honors degrees, but still have a chip on my shoulder and a sense of injustice done. I feel to this day the shame of having been branded a failure and that blow to my self-respect has been both a spur to higher endeavor as well as a nagging source of insecurity. I strongly suspect that Miss Jones, in her eighties when I knew her, had a similar chip on the shoulder to mine, for her qualifications were way beyond what were expected of a teacher in a Secondary Modern School. It might account for her ferocity. The quarter of the population of Pontypridd who had been taught by her continued to be scared stiff of her, as were also some of her former colleagues. Why had she not taught in the Grammar School? Local politics, I shouldn't wonder. She was one of those rare teachers who could teach any subject under the sun and her range included calculus and classical Greek. After retirement she continued to give coaching to those brave enough to spend an hour in her company in her Edwardian drawing room. On one occasion I had cause to visit Miss Jones on some item of church business. She had just dismissed one of her students who she had sent away with a flea in his ear. "I told him I had no intention of teaching him until he got his hair cut." "Miss Jones", I said, "you are an enthusiastic supporter of the Liberal Party?" "Indeed," she replied, "I was ward secretary for many years." "Did you ever meet Lloyd George?" I asked. Her bosom visibly swelled with pride as she said, "I was privileged to share the same platform with him on many occasions." "What did you think of him?" "He was the greatest Prime Minister this country has ever known." I paused for the kill. "Miss Jones, how did Lloyd George wear his hair?" Chware teg, as we say in Wales, she took the point. (Chware teg = 'fair play').

It is amazing how steamed up people can be even today in the twenty-first century over the length of somebody else's hair. It's amazing that in our much vaunted pluralistic and permissive society that such an item should have any importance whatsoever. I sometimes wear a kilt (a Welsh tartan) and you can always count on someone to make a silly remark. In the days of Jesus, long hair in a male was a mark of holiness, perhaps because someone who did not attend to their hair might be considered to have their mind on higher things. Today the same feature is either the mark of the artistic temperament, of the alternative life style, or the gentler type of yob. (The word 'holy' means 'different', so perhaps nothing has changed) It is still more respectable for a man to have short back and sides, and his chances at an interview will be seriously in jeopardy if he does not comply. Sometimes prejudice can be adjusted to make way for other considerations, as in the case of Miss Jones. Funny how Jesus is never criticized for having long hair! Jesus' brother James calls the Christians of his day to ignore outward appearance in their dealings with other people.

My friends, those who are true followers of our great-hearted Leader, Jesus The Chosen One, don't display snobbery. Suppose someone wearing expensive jewelry and clothes comes into your meeting, and someone poor, wearing dirty clothes, comes in at the same time. If you pay special attention to the one who's well-dressed... you're being snobbish and judging on the basis of prejudice.

('The Call to Action' 2:3)

On one occasion Paul got his hair cut before setting out on a journey. Some translations seem to suggest that he cut his hair in order to indicate his vow. This may be the origin of the tonsure in Christian monastic tradition, the practice, less common nowadays, of monks or nuns shaving their heads as a sign that they are bound by vows. Almost certainly this is a misunderstanding. Paul's haircut marked the end of his vow not the beginning, since it was long hair and not short hair that indicated dedication to God, as with Samson in the book of 'Judges'. The vow may have been one of abstinence from meat or strong drink or sex – all three forms of abstinence are to be found in the Hebrew scriptures- or something more positive such as extra prayer or alms giving for a period. It always helps to read scripture texts in context. The fact that Paul handed over his missionary work to Cill and Will in Ephesus may simply mean that Paul had completed a timed stint of evangelism and was now going to have a break. Very sensible – Dr. Luke's orders perhaps. However, it should come as a bit of a shock that Paul bothered at all about outward shows of piety, especially if he shared Luke's knowledge of the teaching of Jesus. Luke alone of the gospel writers records the parable of Jesus that contrasts the outward display of righteousness on the part of the member of the strict set – "I keep to a strict diet, and I give generously to charity" and the inner sorrow of the tax collector, looked on as a traitor and an outcast from society, "God help me. I'm no good!" (1Luke 18:9) Perhaps Luke is giving a gentle tap on the knuckles to the man who considered himself to be no longer under the law but under grace. The whole question arises of the practice of Christians, maybe on the basis of Paul, but against the strong advice and example of Jesus, of wearing special clothing to identify themselves. (Matthew 23:5) This applies not only to all ranks of clergy who have gone at it with a will, but also to the rest of Christians many of whom can be identified quite easily when they are on their way to church by what they are wearing, and sometimes by their hairstyles. Christians should practice the art of holy invisibility. We will be identified soon enough when the need arises, by our kindness.

FORESKIN

Paul went on to Derby and then Lester. Lester was where Timothy lived. He was a new Christian. His mother was Jewish and his father Greek. His mother was a Christian too. Timothy was popular with the Christians in those parts. Paul asked Timothy to join his team. Paul cut off Timothy's foreskin to please the Jews who lived in the area. They suspected Timothy had not had this done to him earlier because his father was Greek. In every town they visited, they told the Christians about the guidelines agreed by the leading Christians in Jerusalem. 2Luke 16:1.

Eluned Jones, headmistress of Cardiff High School in the days I taught history there, a stalwart of Bethany Baptist Church Rhiwbina, and an encourager of my preaching, said on hearing an extract from the draft of this book, "You're just out to debunk, John." I suppose that is an understandable reflex reaction. Some of my friends suggested that the very title *Bad Acts of the Apostles* was offensively provocative, and that I should resort to some such title as 'The Church steps out'. Those friends knew nothing about selling books. An arresting title is the first prerequisite if your book is going to sell. Anyone who takes the trouble to read what I have written will realize that I have a higher purpose in mind than debunking anybody. My aim is to champion Jesus as our leader and example. Another friend called this work 'a subversive little book'. I hope so, if by that is meant a book that joins with a much needed wider movement to subvert those powers and authorities who have pushed Jesus out of his central place. Although debunking (or subverting) has not been my prime intention, I would suggest that debunking and subverting is good for Christians of every generation, especially for leaders. If we get knocked off our pedestals the answer is that we should not have been standing on them in the first place. I think the first Christian leaders would agree. That is not to say that they, any more than ourselves, would find the experience of being criticized easy to cope with. However, they regarded themselves as friends of Jesus and had no idea of setting themselves up as a secondary authority to his. He was the only authority, and his the only standard by which any action or attitude might be judged. If they could be shown, as Rocky was shown at Jaffa, that any behavior of theirs had been untrue to Jesus, they accepted the criticism and endeavored to change their ways. They did this sometimes reluctantly, sometimes with difficulty, but they knew it was what their leader expected of them. Moreover, the religious movement in which they played so prominent a part was anything but a new set of tablets from Mount Sinai. It was a movement propelled by the Spirit who blew where she wished. Situations rapidly developed calling for constant adaptation, and the leaders made many of their decisions on the hoof, confirming some and regretting others, but constantly moving on, looking for the next challenge, the next call to bold and radical thought. They disagreed, fell out and were reconciled again. The idea that faith in the sense of a religious system can be built upon the 'apostles' is ludicrous and blasphemous. It denies the sense of dynamism and movement that was their experience, and robs the risen Jesus of his authority. What we need to take from these pioneers is their spirit of adventure, not their decisions which were situational nor their organization which was ad hoc. This way of looking at things will be disturbing or annoying to Christians who like to use the label 'apostolic' for their particular brand of Gnostic elitism, just as intelligent study of the Bible affronts those who use the label 'bible-believer' for the same purpose.

The bricklayer must be careful to build up from the foundation already in place. No one should try to replace it with another. The foundation is Jesus, God's Chosen.(1Corinthians 3:11)

These studies suggest that Luke in recording the doings of the first Christian leaders provides us with a running appraisal of their performance. There is no doubt that his main purpose was to inspire future generations to the highest of actions in the name of Jesus. As part of this purpose it is possible to detect critical notes, sometimes intended, sometimes perhaps unconscious. There is a tinge of anxiety in the text and the withholding of comment at critical stages. We can be quite sure he was not congratulating the leaders when he recorded their disputes. But neither could he congratulate them when, as sometimes he must have realized, they contradicted in their behavior what he had learnt from his researches to be the mind and manner of Jesus. Sometimes he might have been blind to those contradictions due to his involvement and absorption in the events. But in striving to provide us with an honest account he has given us the tools to be critical and we will not be out of step with him if sometimes we come down on the side of an unfavorable judgment. I believe if we could have a face to face with Luke today he would open the text and point to instances overlooked in these studies, and have the full approval of his first century Christian comrades for so doing.

So we end with an incident that Luke records which almost certainly in his opinion was a bad act, and which was confirmed as such by the repentance of the perpetrator.

Timothy was one of Paul's prize converts. Paul picked him up at Lester on his second missionary journey. He was the sort of convert every evangelist dreams of making, someone with the obvious gifts and qualities that will fit him to assist with the work.

Tim immediately joined Paul's missionary team and stuck with Paul for the rest of his life, often deputizing for Paul when he was unable to visit one of the Christian groups. The picture we get of Tim from the references in Paul's letters, especially from the snippets of genuine Paul in the two otherwise doubtful 'letters to Timothy', is of a shy, retiring young man. The description 'meek' would sum him up. Paul had to warn Tim against allowing himself to be put upon. When Paul sent him to Corinth in his place he wrote:

If Timothy drops in to see you, please make him feel at home. He's working for the Leader as hard as I am. Make sure no-one makes fun of him and that when the time comes for him to leave, he's relaxed for his journey home to me.(1Corinthians 16:10)

We get the impression of a man who did not always assert himself in his own interests. Tim was the child of a mixed marriage, his mother a Jewess and his father a Greek. He followed his father in being uncircumcised, although he shared his mother's religion. Paul regarded it as expedient that Tim have his foreskin removed to be more acceptable to potential Jewish converts, and to this Tim submitted, Paul performing the operation. Luke has a particularly snide way of putting this. Paul did it, he says, because the Jews knew that Tim's father was Greek, as if to say that in other circumstances an uncircumcised companion might pass, since the feature could only be discovered in intimate circumstances. In Tim's case questions were liable to be asked. Without actually saying that a piece of hypocrisy is in progress, Luke gets pretty close. The same kind of hypocrisy is practiced in Christian circles today on the gay issue. Clergy are advised by their superiors that providing they keep their gay orientation hidden by being discreet they have nothing to worry about, but if they should be found out as 'practicing' (including the public taking of a partner) then they will have to be disciplined. We have the ludicrous situation where a gay minister or priest can be promiscuous providing he or she is careful, whereas if he or she sets a good example by being committed and loyal to one person, he/she is in for trouble! A gay person may hide their sexuality by marrying someone of the opposite sex, but if they remain single questions will almost certainly be asked and dishonesty thereby encouraged. It is difficult to avoid the impression that the Church prefers hypocrisy to the truth. Non-Christians are fully aware of the Church's weakness, even if Christians are not. "They're a load of hypocrites" may be an unfair verdict, but it is well grounded.

Luke sets the account of Tim's circumcision almost immediately after the account of the Council of Jerusalem (chapter 15) in which the Christian leaders make it abundantly clear that non-Jews were not to be obliged to submit to circumcision. Paul was therefore out of order. Can it be doubted that Luke sets these two events side by side to emphasize this very point? For a mature man the operation would have been uncomfortable and embarrassing and according to the ideas of the time an affront to his national identity as a Greek. Luke also was Greek. We can almost hear him saying, "He didn't dare try that one on me!" There is no hint of protest from Tim. Humble submission was the essence of his character. All the more reason for Paul to have more respect for him. But enough criticism of Paul! Paul is his own critic and the proof, if we need it, that Luke records bad acts as well as good acts. Paul's letter to the Celtic Christians (Galatians) was written sometime after Tim's circumcision. The greater part of the letter is devoted to condemning those who insist on circumcision. Paul calls them 'dogs'. Most telling of all is Paul's mention of the fact that he did not circumcise Titus despite pressure for this to be done and although Titus was to accompany Paul to Jerusalem. They were going into the lion's den. (2:1-14) No counsel of expediency this time! Paul refers to spies in their group, trying to find out whether Titus was circumcised or not. Following him to the baths and taking a peep? By this time Paul is adamant. There is to be no more losing of foreskins just to please the heavy brigade and he records how he found it necessary to rebuke Rocky for not being sufficiently firm and consistent in the matter.

It is not debunking to criticize the 'apostles'. It is honoring them for their humanity. They criticized one another and they were self-critical. They were on the look out for hypocrisy and double standards. They can help us identify these ills in our time because they sometimes fell prey to them in theirs. Our humanity is one; our shortcomings are the same. We do not honor them and they cannot help us if we insist on giving them halos that rob them of flesh and blood. We can only profit from their example if we also learn from their mistakes.

FOR SPLENDID FOLK

(1) For splendid folk who have gone home to God.
Those who, on earth, life's pavements finely trod,
And whose example gladly we applaud,
Praise to their memory
While still we journey.

(2) You taught them love, its way its truth, its life,
Jesus, God's Likeness, answer to earth's strife;
Reason their tool, replacing fist and knife,
Praise to their memory
While still we journey.

(3) May we, like them, be in our thinking bold,
Leaving behind the patterns worn and old,
Drawn on by wisdom's gleam, not that of gold,
Praise to their memory
While still we journey.

(4) The day will come when we with them unite,
     All in new clothing, colors gay and bright;
     Darkness at last defeated, only light,
          Sharing our memories
          Of all our journeys.

(After W.W.How 1823-97 'For all the Saints')

Chapter Fifteen

LUKE'S APOSTLES

The accusation of Eluned Jones that my volume '*The Bad Acts of the Apostles*' is a debunking exercise continues to play on my mind, since the object of all my writing is to present a positive and joyful version of the Good News. Indeed I consider those forms of Christianity that put an emphasis on wrongdoings and on what a wicked world we live in, and even present the cross as exclusively to do with sin and God's disapproval, do not merit the description 'Good News' or 'Evangelical'. Have I fallen into the same trap? To be a Good News Christian you must avoid belly aching. However, some elements of the belly aching, that is to say 'bad news' aspects of Christianity, began with the very first Christian leaders when they fell short of the example and teaching of their Leader Jesus. I have felt drawn to accompany Luke as he pinpoints these aspects so that Good News Christians can avoid being bearers of bad news in the future.

Luke provides us with a penetrating appraisal of the performance of the early Church. That must have been his intention and not just accidental, for Luke reveals himself to be a skilful, subtle and ingenious writer with a great and noble mind. In thinking about Luke's intentions, we cannot avoid negative territory. Luke would have been upset by the Church's title for the second part of his work, as would the author of a book on cordon bleu recipes if the publisher had presented it with the title, 'Guides to Easy Cooking'. The title 'The Acts of the Apostles' is irresponsibly misleading. J.B. Phillips, in his ground-breaking translation of the Christian scriptures styled the work, 'The Young Church in Action', which supplies the gentle hint, if you think about it, that the Church portrayed therein still had much to learn. Eugene

Peterson in his valuable and bouncy version 'The Message' demonstrates an awareness of the issue by calling the book "The Acts", leaving his readers to find out whose acts. These 'acts' are certainly not those of the twelve apostles as traditionally understood. Luke provides us near the start with a list of the names of Jesus' associates, identical with that in his first volume (6:13), but interestingly not in quite the same order. We get the impression from both lists that the front runners appear at the beginning and the also-rans towards the end. In volume two the list seems more open in that the women friends of Jesus are mentioned in the very next breath and not positioned separately as in Luke's first volume (8:2). This time the sole woman to be identified by name is Mary the mother of Jesus who appears as a member of the disciple group for the first (and last) time. Jesus' brothers also get a mention, but not by name. The only people on this list whose acts are subsequently recorded in 'The Acts' are those of Rocky and John. The execution of John's brother Jim is recorded without any account of his contribution to the life of the community. John only appears as a companion of Rocky. This means that of the official list of 'apostles' only Rocky is given any kind of prominence or character sketch. However Jesus' brother James does appear again more than once. He is portrayed as having an important role, seeming to wield the influence and authority of an 'apostle'. Maybe after the death of Jim Zebedee, James the brother of Jesus stepped into his namesake's shoes to make up the number twelve again, as Matthias did by means of a lottery. Or maybe this James was held in awe simply because he was Jesus' brother and resembled him in looks.

This begs the question as to how significant the list of 'twelve' apostles is, if at all. Michael Ball believes the twelve were appointed by Jesus with the restricted brief of addressing the Good News to their own Jewish people. That is where their authority and their activity very largely began and ended. They mirrored the sons of Jacob who gave their names to the 'twelve tribes of Israel'. Here were twelve new names to mark the commencement of a new covenant and a renewed people of God. My own view is that we should understand that for the most part the numbers given in the scriptures are to be understood as symbolic. The numbers 3, 7 and 12 in particular are regarded as special or holy. It is unlikely there were exactly 'twelve' tribes of Israel. Joseph's tribe had to be divided into two to cook the numbers when the tribe of Levi was set apart for priestly duties. There was also possibly a Kenite tribe deriving from Moses' father-in-law and a tribe deriving from Dinah, Jacob's daughter, as well as smaller tribes, such as the Gibeonites, who though looked down on were included. The lists of the 'apostles' in the Synoptic gospels (Mark, Matthew and Luke) are not exactly the same. Mark and Matthew include Thaddaeus whereas Luke has an extra Judas 'the son of James' (he does not tell us which James). 'Sources Close' (John's Gospel) hardly mentions the concept of the 'twelve' and has no list. But if we draw up a list from the mention of key disciples, it is a very different list from the other gospels. It consists of (in order of appearance):-Andrew + another (his wife or intended? – disciples of John the Dipper, wearing camel skins like their teacher perhaps); Rocky, Philip, Nathan (Nathanael), Nick (Nicodemus), Samantha (the Samaritan woman – according to this gospel, Andrew was the first evangelist, Samantha the second!); Larry (Lazarus), Mary and Martha; Twin (Thomas); two called Judas (one from Kerioth, one not); 'another' – known to the high priest- his concubine possibly (we are looking for someone intimate with Guy, but a secret disciple of Jesus. A court concubine would fit the bill.); Jesus' aunt Miriam (Clover's wife), Maggie (Mary Magdala), Joseph from Ram; 'the sons of Zebedee' i.e. Jim and John, and one of 'two others' who go out fishing (the other one being identified as Jesus' special friend i.e. Larry). The other 'other' is a real mystery, but in view of Rocky's nudity in the story almost certainly male, unless – a long shot - it turns out to be Rocky's wife. I make that 18. No doubt you will quarrel with this list and call my guesses wild, but start leaving people out to get the number down to 12 and I am sure you will also disagree among yourselves. You might manage it by leaving the women out, which is how the other gospel writers managed to hold the numbers down to about twelve. The author of 'Sources Close' does at least give us thumbnail sketches of most of these disciples, whereas Matthew, Mark and Luke seem to know very little about most of the people on their lists. (Incidentally an important point for those, like myself, who ascribe 'Sources Close' an early date.) The tail-enders on the official lists fade into the mists. Later Christian communities were obliged to invent traditions for them, generally highly dubious and unconvincing, as improbable as the bones produced as evidence. Did Luke know anything about who they were or their stories? We have to conclude that these good folk, friends of Jesus though they must have been, made so little impact on the story of the early Christian community that Luke thinks there is nothing sufficiently exciting to tell us about them nor indeed about Matthias, the faceless replacement as number 12.

After he has sent most of the 'twelve' to oblivion, Luke sets about telling us who were the real leaders in the early Church. He would have rejected the title 'Acts of the Apostles' for his narrative, but he might have given the thumbs up to 'The Acts of the Alternative Apostles.' These were people who took the Good News both to Jews and non- Jews as well as to other classes of outsider. According to Luke, Rocky alone of the 'twelve' appointed by Jesus handed on the Good News to a Gentile, though the author of 'Sources Close' tells us that Andrew and Philip brought some Greeks to Jesus. Who were the true apostles according to Luke? They were Rocky, Steven, Philip the Good News Seller, Gazelle (Dorcas), Paul, Ian (Ananias), Cheery (Barnabas), Mark, Silas, Lydia, Ray (Apollos) and the duo Cill and Will (Priscilla and Acquila) That makes a dozen if we count Cill and Will together, a baker's dozen if we count them separately! We would probably vote to add Luke's name to the list, but he would probably not wish to vote for himself. There are more than twelve characters in 'Acts' who inspire Luke's respect and admiration, the fortune-teller of Philiptown, for example. You can alter or add to the list to suit yourself. The apostles in the official listings are conspicuous by their absence, with the exception of Rocky.

I want to end this volume by having a look at these alternative apostles. No one can deny that they are Luke's heroes. He gives Rocky and Paul most prominence and we get good, honest, realistic portraits of these two spiritual and human giants. They do very good things and very bad things, just like us. But without them it is difficult to imagine Christianity ever becoming a European, then world-wide religion. The precept, useful at times, 'No-one is indispensable' is not true with God. God enjoys depending on a certain number of prize characters (only God knows them all) who give everything they've got to the New World Project, their weaknesses as well as their strengths, their badness as well as their goodness. For Luke, undoubtedly Rocky's very best act was his acknowledgement of Neil, the Roman Centurion, as a man of God before his conversion, and as a brother in Christ afterwards. This required a difficult and agonizing remaking of Rocky himself, a traumatic experience that obliged him to jettison his deep-seated and ugly prejudices. Saints are those who permit themselves to be shaken to the very foundations of their most treasured and assured beliefs in order to be more surely founded on Jesus. Rocky's worst act through the eyes of Luke was his treatment of Nye and Sapphire. Luke removes Rocky's halo and portrays him as a sinner, which is what every true saint is found on closer examination to be. As for Paul, his worst act was his inhumanity towards Slippery Al. His best and greatest act was his plea for freedom on behalf of his Gentile converts at the Jerusalem council, supported by Rocky and James.

Without Paul Christianity would have become a denomination within Judaism. Some Christians are just that, since they have in reality rejected the teachings of Paul with regard to freedom from the Law and trust in Christ alone.

But significantly, not alongside Rocky and Paul, but prior to them in terms of time, Luke presents two other major heroes. The time sequence is crucial and Luke quite deliberately demonstrates that without the work of Steven and Philip the Good News Monger, the great work of Rocky and Paul might not have happened.

Steven

The connection between the martyrdom of Steven and the conversion of Saul (later Paul) is well-trodden ground. Paul's conversion, recounted by Luke and by Paul himself twice to make three times in 'Acts', was an event that affected the deepest caverns of his being. He was changed, almost in a moment, it would seem, from being an unpleasant, heartless, persecuting bigot into a warm-hearted, caring, lover of Jesus and all humanity. Of course, it was not as quick as that, - no true conversion ever is. There is an in-the-womb period to every conversion, and also a never ending period of adjustment and growth afterwards. Steven was undoubtedly an important stage in the coming to birth of the new Paul, as was also Paul's observation of the behavior of other Christians at the receiving end of his harassment. Paul it seems did not throw a stone at Steven, but he was all in favor of it and looked after the coats of the executioners. According to Luke Paul was 'consenting' to Steven's death, but one wonders why he opted to be cloak attendant rather than an active participant. Was his holding back a sign that something was already happening to him? Usually he was a leader, setting an example, so why did he not throw the first stone on this occasion? Standing apart gave him the opportunity to observe intently, to watch Steven's face and to hear his prayer for forgiveness on his enemies. Paul was a spiritual person and the sight of someone praying calmly and lovingly under such conditions, must have affected him greatly. The teaching of Paul on non-retaliation and love for our enemies must owe something to Steven's example, as well as to the example of Jesus himself. Paul was not there at the cross, but for him the courageous and forgiving death of Steven must have served as a re-enactment.

There is more to this than the stirring of Paul's emotions. Steven was brought before the Jewish council to answer for his 'heresies' and Paul was there to hear him, either as a member of the council himself or as an observer. Luke quotes Steven's speech (more like a sermon) in full. Someone must have taken notes. Or were Steven's words so imprinted on Paul's memory that he was able to repeat them later to Luke, almost word for word. That presumes an intense listening on the part of Paul and an intense state of mind. Some observers noted that Steven 'had the face of an angel'. Was Paul one of these observers? Was Steven a particularly good looking young man? Or was it just his bright smile that half attracted, half annoyed the assembled clergy? If Paul mentally put Steven's speech on disc, he had much to think about for some while to come.

Steven gave an account of the history of the ancestors of the Jewish people. He certainly knew the scriptures. There were several recurring themes which Steven emphasized and used to make the points he hoped would convince but in the event infuriated his audience. Every preacher worth their salt has had this experience sometime or another. The more convincing you are, the less they like it! Donald Soper said of preaching, "You must put it twice as strongly as you mean, because they are only half listening!" Steven's audience couldn't help listening or getting the message- it was only too clear.

The Jewish patriarchs were mobile not static. Abraham moved from Ur to Canaan; Joseph moved to Egypt; Moses moved from Egypt to the desert and led his compatriots to the Promised Land.

This theme of mobility leads Steven on to the question of the place of worship. A mobile people following a mobile God required a tent which could be taken down and put up somewhere else. The temple was a mistake and Steven quoted texts expressing God's disapproval. Another theme Steven developed was the involvement of God's ancient people with people of other races. Abraham bought the land for his tomb from the Hamor family in Samaria; Joseph was the Egyptian Pharaoh's Prime Minister; Moses was brought up by Pharaoh's daughter. Steven's third theme was the rebelliousness and stubbornness of God's people throughout their history, forever thwarting God's purposes and killing God's special messengers. Finally Steven said, *"They killed those who said God's special messenger was coming, and now you've murdered him by handing him over to the enemy! You've been told what God wants of you by God's messengers. But you've done the opposite!"* (7:53) Steven was allowed to say no more, but he had said enough to set Saul, as he was then, on several trains of thought. Being God's person and a dyed-in-the-wool traditionalist are incompatible. God moves, so must you. God works in cooperation with people of all faiths and lifestyles, so must you. Reject the love shown in Jesus and copied faithfully by his disciple Steven, and you reject God. All this surfaced again in the teaching of Paul after it had had time to ferment. Paul stalked out of the synagogue more than once and conducted his meetings in borrowed rooms, houses or in the open air. He was a mobile Christian, fond of the metaphor of the athlete to describe the Christian life. He learned to get alongside Gentiles of all types and conditions and classes from the very high to the very low. He set forth the cross as the central point of his preaching, and the quality love shown at Calvary as the goal for the Jesus person.

Luke shows us that Paul was not the first great theologian of the Christian Church. That honor must go to Steven. He was not a minor prophet. He provided the thinking, based on an educated and imaginative understanding of the scriptures, which was to bring into being a mobile, inclusive and loving people. Not all would go his way, or Paul's. But there would be enough to keep the flame burning.

The Son of God adventures out

The Son of God adventures out
A hero's fame to win;
His rainbow banner waves aloft,
Who dares to follow him?
Who dares to drink his offered cup
With love filled to the brim?
Who dares to take a rough cross up?
Who dares to follow him?

Steven it was whose angel eye
Could pierce beyond the grave;
He saw his leader in the sky
And called on him to save;
Like Jesus, pardon on his tongue,
As murderers crowded in,
He prayed for those who did the wrong;
Who dares to follow him?

Courageous band, at first a few,
On whom the Spirit came;
Brave or alarmed, their hope they knew,
And mocked the cross and flame.
They faced the angry soldier's steel
And in the lion's den
They bowed their necks the death to feel;
Who dares to follow them?

Eternal friends, from every strand
Of rich humanity,
They now around their leader stand,
A merry company;
They climbed the steep ascent of heaven
Through peril, pain and sin;
Dear God, may love to us be given
Who dare to follow them.

(After Reginald Heber 1783-1826. The Son of God goes forth to war.)

Philip the Good News Seller

Philip was a colleague of Steven's among the 'lower ranks' of the first Christian clergy. If he were around at the time, he would have been one of the young men who attended to Steven's burial. Like Steven he was a radical who 'did his own thing' under the direct guidance of God's Spirit. Luke gives him a position of prominence by recording his mission to Samaria; to Africa by means of his conversion of one of the Ethiopian Queen's gay courtiers; to the Philistines of the coastal regions; and not so often remarked upon, to the Gentile centre of Caesartown. This was where Rocky was to convert and dip Neil, the Roman Centurion. In a small town by our standards, we must regard it as most unlikely that Philip did not meet Neil prior to Rocky's visit at Neil's invitation. It was well known that Neil was a good man and a seeker after God, though by culture and nurture a pagan. He would have been a prime target for Philip, who we can imagine using the same technique as he used with the Ethiopian. Philip would have relied on his knowledge of the scriptures and fitted them to Neil's case. Perhaps he would have told Neil about Norman the Syrian, a worshipper of Rimon, who found the true God by visiting Elis, God's Speaker and having a dip in the river Jordan. Luke tells us that Neil was visited by a messenger from God. Traditional translations use the word 'angel', but the Greek 'angelos' means 'messenger' or 'helper'. Because of the persistent, now misleading, translation of the word as 'angel', we immediately in our mind's eye see a sexually ambivalent android with wings. Angels were not portrayed with wings until the Middle Ages. Because Luke uses 'angelos' when he indicates a special messenger from God, readers of his two volumes conclude that he had a special interest in supernatural beings. Maybe he did. But it is more likely that Luke thought that angels were usually humans who give God a helping hand. That is what angels are for the most part in the Bible, apart from the apocalyptic writings (Daniel, Revelation etc). So Philip must be a very good candidate for the 'angel' who recommended to Neil that he send for Rocky. A regular feature of Luke's 'angels', probably human, is that they appeared suddenly on the scene and left just as suddenly, like the prophets in the Hebrew scriptures. This was true of the messenger called Gabriel who came to Mary; the angel who strengthened Jesus in the garden near the olive press; and the angel who helped Rocky escape from prison. Luke's 'helping hands' quickly got off the scene when they had done their work, enabling their charges to stand on their own feet and avoid continual dependence on others. Philip fits this pattern. He did not linger with the Ethiopian to supervise his future spiritual progress. He quickly made himself scarce.

Philip's visit to Neil was angelically brief. He dropped his crucial message, then flitted off again. From now on he would not interfere but let God's Spirit and another of her servants get on with the job. When Philip's work of outreach in Samaria had required an official stamp of approval as well as a bit of encouragement, the visit of Rocky and John fitted the bill. Instead of waiting this time for Rocky or some other apostle to catch up with him and tick him off for stepping out of line, Philip arranged for an apostle to preside over the next big leap forward for the Gospel. This was slick thinking on his part. The fact that Neil responded to the preaching of Rocky rather than to the preaching of Philip, and was dipped by Rocky too, meant that the authority of an undisputed companion of Jesus was to certify the inclusion of a prominent Gentile from the ranks of the Roman conquerors into the Christian Church. This step was to prove highly controversial and it needed all Rocky's authority to get it accepted, including his assurance of proof positive that Neil and all his household - family, servants and friends - had received the gift of the Spirit. An even more intriguing possibility is that Philip visited Rocky on his way to Caesartown. Jaffa was on route from Azotus. He may have chatted at length with Rocky about his successes with the Ethiopian and the ancient Philistine towns and prepared Rocky mentally for his dream/vision on the rooftop of his lodgings at Simon the Tanner's. Thus Philip may have had some responsibility for the spiritual preparation of both Rocky and Neil. It would have been much easier for the first century Christians than for us, as they read Luke's account, to follow in their mind's eye the tracks of Rocky and Philip, because this was their land and they knew the geography. We cannot work out what was going on unless it occurs to us to consult a map.

As a Baptist, though I do not accept the authority of bishops as such, I accept the authority of the wise leadership, intellect, experience and expertise which some of my friends who are bishops abundantly display. I have found bishops helpful on occasion for pushing God's work forward by dint of the fact that they just happen to be bishops. As a teenager in the 1950s I was a member of my father's church in Southmead, Bristol, set in the middle of a large and problem ridden housing estate. The churches worked well together and I was an enthusiastic attender at ecumenical events. At a planning meeting the question was raised of an ecumenical Communion Service. The Anglican vicar immediately brought the discussion to an end by saying sharply, "I'm afraid the bishop would not allow it." At that time I was also a student at Bristol Cathedral School, working for my 'A' levels. A few days later I waylaid Bishop Cockin in the cloisters that adjoined both Cathedral and school. "I'm sorry that we don't have your permission for an ecumenical communion service in Southmead" I said, cheekily. "What's this?" The Bishop visibly bristled. "I'm not in the habit of refusing permission for such requests. I wish I had more of them!" When I told him the circumstances, he said, "Leave it to me!" Straightway he phoned the unfortunate vicar and gave him an earful. We had our ecumenical communion. Sometimes lowly Christians have to step back and get the high flyers to do the job. Philip knew that in the case of such a high profile candidate for conversion as Neil, it required someone of Rocky's stature to handle the inevitable uproar. Rocky was spiritually prepared for the great leap forward. But even Rocky failed to convince all his critics, and battle lines were drawn. The battle continues unabated today on very much the same lines. Luke makes sure that Rocky does not get all the credit. Philip, not Rocky, was the true pioneer. An apostle needed someone to be an apostle to him, to get him moving!

The angel Philip was probably there when Rocky preached in Neil's house and when Neil's capacious bath suite was turned into a baptistry. I suspect Philip hovered in the background, a big smile on his face. Knowing Rocky as we do it is unlikely he invited Philip to take part in the service or acknowledged Philip's share in the great leap forward. But when Rocky had moved on, Philip seems to have settled down in Caesartown to become a family man with wife and four gifted daughters. Does this mean Philip became the accepted leader of the church at Caesartown? Probably – one of the leaders, at least. Did he sometimes share a chuckle with his friend Neil over how they and the Spirit managed to get Rocky on board in the business of winning Gentiles?

Gazelle

In Jaffa there was a friend of Jesus whose name was Gazelle. She was always helping other people, especially poor people. At this time she had a serious illness and died. Her body was laid in a room upstairs. Ludd was not far away, so when the Christians in Jaffa heard Rocky was there, they sent two messengers to him, asking him to come as soon as possible. Rocky packed his belongings and went straight back with them to Jaffa. When he got there he was taken upstairs straightaway. Some poor women were in the bedroom. They crowded round Rocky and showed him the coats and dresses Gazelle had made while she was alive.Rocky sent everybody out of the room. Then he knelt beside the bed and talked with God. He looked at the body and said, "Come on, Gazelle, it's time to get up!" Gazelle opened her eyes, and when she saw Rocky, she sat up. Rocky held her hand as she got out of bed. Then he called for the other friends to come up, including the women who had been there. He showed them that Gazelle was alive. Soon everyone in Jaffa was talking about what had happened, and many put their trust in Jesus. Rocky stayed on in Jaffa, lodging with a leather-maker called Simon.(9: 36)

It is difficult to avoid the conclusion that Luke, of all the gospel writers, was the champion of women. He certainly was, though the other gospel writers championed women too in their own way. Matthew, for example, includes some prominent and interesting women in his list of Jesus' ancestors. Luke did not add to the ministry of Jesus an aspect that was not there, crafting Jesus in his own image. The special concern of Jesus for women, and his radical inclusion of them on his team, is witnessed in all the gospels, and if we did not possess Luke, we could still pick up on it. Luke continued to champion women in his second volume, which, as we have seen, was written side by side with volume one. His first female hero/apostle was a friend of Jesus with the beautiful name Gazelle, the meaning of 'Tabitha' in Aramaic and 'Dorcas' in Greek. Today Tabitha or Dorcas are still sometimes chosen as a Christian name for a girl, but without appreciation for the original feel of the name. We even call a cat 'Tabitha' without reflecting that gazelles are hunted and killed by big cats! Since

Gazelle had been a friend of Jesus during his ministry, we are bound to wonder whether it was the name given to her by her parents, or whether it was a nickname given to her by Jesus as an expression of her character, like the nickname Rocky given to Simon Johnson. The description 'friend of Jesus', which we use in Good As New, in the Greek text is a feminine version of the word 'disciple', the word Luke uses of the 'twelve' male disciples (1Luke 8:9 also Matthew 10:1) Our discovery that Gazelle had been on Jesus' team must lead us to suspect that the scant references to women disciples in the gospels by name is not a true reflection of the number of women friends Jesus had with him. There were more, perhaps many more. The confidence with which the Christians of Jaffa sent to Rocky with news of Gazelle's illness, and the ready willingness with which Rocky rushed to get to her, gives us some idea of her status among the first friends of Jesus. There are women in the gospels whose names we are not given but who bore witness to the events of the death and coming to life of Jesus. Most likely Gazelle was one of these. It seems Gazelle had, like Rocky, and many others, fled north into Gentile territory to escape persecution. In Jaffa she had set up a house of refuge for the poor women of the town. She had made a great impression and was loved not only by the women she had helped, but by the whole community. She was gifted as a dressmaker, and put this talent to good use in her work of charity.

Rocky brought Gazelle back to full life and health. The way it happened provides further evidence that they knew each other well. Gazelle recognized Rocky's voice and when she opened her eyes she recognized his face and sat up. Then Rocky held her hand as she got out of bed, another sign of their intimacy. It's the kind of physical gesture Jesus confidently made to women, without hesitation, despite the fact that men were not supposed to touch women, unless they were family. Rocky was instinctively or deliberately copying the behavior of Jesus, perhaps remembering the way Jesus had brought back Jay's daughter from the point of death.

We do not need to be ace theologians to work out why Luke puts Gazelle among his apostle team. It does not depend on any status she had from knowing Jesus as a friend, or from being a witness to the resurrection. It is because she was an example of what being a true follower of Jesus is all about. It is not to do with power and authority, but with service. The words Luke quotes Jesus as saying at the Last Supper, Jesus must have spoken on many other occasions, for Mark records it at a different point. In any case, Gazelle probably got the message by watching Jesus just as much as by hearing his words:

Jesus said, "You know how many countries have leaders who bully their subjects, despite calling themselves 'friends of the people'. You must not imitate them. Anyone who wants an important role must humbly seek the advice and experience of others, and anyone who thinks they have leadership qualities must show they are not above doing the dirty jobs. The needs of the customers in a restaurant come before the needs of the waiter. I'm showing you how to act like the perfect waiter."(1Luke 22: 25)

In the story Luke tells of Rocky and Gazelle he paints portraits of two apostles in one picture. Which apostle was most like Jesus?

Ian

In Damascus there was a friend of Jesus called Ian. He had a dream in which Jesus spoke to him by name. 'What is it, Leader?" he asked.Jesus said, "Go to Jude's house in Straight Street, and ask for a man from Tarsus called Saul. He is spending his time talking with God. He's dreamt that someone called Ian will come and touch him, so he can see again."Ian said, "Leader, I've heard a lot about this man. He's been big trouble to your people in Jerusalem. He's come here with warrants from the clergy to arrest anyone who uses your name in worship." But Jesus said to him, "It's safe for you to go. I've picked this person to be my representative to those who are not Jews. He will act as my ambassador to heads of state. He'll speak for me to his own Jewish people too. I'll have to warn him about all the suffering he'll get when he stands up for me."

Ian made his way to the house and went inside. He hugged Saul and said, "Saul, my friend, Jesus our Leader, the one you met on the way here, has asked me to visit you. You're going to be able to see again, and you'll be filled with God's Spirit." At once the film over Saul's eyes began to clear, and he could see again He got up and was dipped. After having something to eat, he began to feel stronger. Saul spent a few days with the followers of Jesus in Damascus. He started straightaway to speak in the places of worship, saying, "Jesus is God's Likeness." (9,10).

On one occasion I was one of a team of ministers leading an ecumenical study group. We decided on 'The friends of Paul' as our theme. The other members were surprised when I offered to introduce 'Ananias' for my turn. "No, you don't understand, John" they said, "Ananias was not a friend of Paul, simply someone who helped him on one occasion.""I call that a friend," I said. I stuck to my guns and hope I convinced. I was remembering an experience I had at the start of my breakdown when I was not very 'with it' at all. I was confined to my home and refused to receive visits from anyone, including my best friends. I hardly came out of my bedroom where I insisted on the blind being drawn at all times. One day I must have been feeling a bit better, for Valerie had persuaded me to come down downstairs and sit in the lounge. There was a knock on the door and I started at once to go to pieces. Before I had time to do anything about it, Valerie had shown in Revd. Gordon Roberts, of all people. Gordon Roberts was the arch-fundamentalist among the clergy of Pontypridd. He was greatly feared, for he rebuked sinners to their faces, and was not known for a bedside manner of pastoral counseling. But I have to say that his visit was a model of how a pastor should be on such an occasion. He did not quote texts, he did not pray over me, he did not, as far as I can recall say anything of a religious nature whatsoever, and he did not stay long. I felt very much better after his visit, and indeed made an important step on the way to recovery. Gordon was a true friend. I only ever saw him again once. It was on a bus and excitedly he told me his son was going in for the Baptist ministry. Gordon was a Presbyterian. He did not seem to mind his son switching. He was pleased as punch! Gordon was an Ananias to me, and I have never forgotten or ceased to be grateful.

We know next to nothing about Ananias – 'Ian' in Good As New. But I love guessing. There are three people called Ananias in Luke's second volume. We give them different names in Good As New in order to avoid confusion. But we may see here another example of Luke's use of the special number 3. The other two were 'baddies'. Ian is the one in the middle, the 'goodie'. He shares the name Ananias with a high priest, a notoriously nasty piece of work, and with the married man from the middle-classes with money to spare. Names are often a class thing. You do not come across many Peregrines among the lower income groups. He may have been a native of Damascus, or a fugitive from Jerusalem. My guess is that he was elderly and a convert to the Jesus 'Way' from the priestly classes, even perhaps an ex-priest. He had almost certainly known Jesus in the flesh and probably was also a witness to the Resurrection. The experience of Jesus speaking to him audibly in his home would count as a Resurrection experience. It was in the same category as Saul's experience on the road and on other occasions. Ian recognized Jesus' voice straightaway, suggesting that he had heard it many times before. *"What is it, Leader?"* Ian had a well-established personal relationship with Jesus and had absolutely no need to clear what he was about to do for Saul with the apostles or indeed with any other Christian. He was naturally nervous and wary of Saul, but also confident and competent in that he had received his instructions directly from Jesus. Like Philip, he did not hesitate to dip someone who many other Christians would regard as a highly questionable candidate for the ceremony. Bringing Saul on board was a risky and radical step.

I am put in mind of the story of Dirk Willems. He was one of the early Anabaptist martyrs. The Anabaptists were radical Protestants and cruelly persecuted on the continent of Europe in the sixteenth and seventeenth centuries. They were the forerunners of the Mennonites, the Amish, the Quakers and the Baptists. A prisoner awaiting execution in the Netherlands, Dirk escaped through a window. He was pursued by one of the prison guards. Light of weight due to his imprisonment, Dirk crossed the thin ice of a pond to safety. His heavier pursuer fell beneath the ice and Dirk turned back and rescued him. The guard took charge of Dirk again, and Dirk was burnt at the stake shortly after. In helping Saul, Ian took the same kind of personal risk. The only thing Ian knew about Saul was that he was a ruthless persecutor of Christians. Was his conversion a trick? Even though it was Jesus who spoke to him, Ian had to ask the question. As it was, Ian was sure to get into trouble with his fellow Christians. Ian was an apostle. Like Maggie, he was an apostle to an apostle to be. We do not know whether Saul/Paul ever met him again. Perhaps not. Perhaps he died soon after, his great work done. Some people only do one big thing for God. That's all God asks of them. Perhaps they do not even notice they are doing it. But their one act is worth another's life's work in effectiveness. There are many types of friend, but the friend who helps out on one critical occasion deserves the accolade 'friend' as much as any other.
('Luke's Apostles' – continued in chapters 16 & 17)

Chapter Sixteen

Luke's Apostles (Continued)

Cheery

Those who accepted the Christian message were a very united group of people. They shared all their belongings and kept nothing for their private use. The leaders spoke with great conviction from their firsthand knowledge that Jesus had returned to life, and everybody felt good. No one went short of anything, because those who owned property put it up for sale and gave the money to the leaders who used it to help anyone in need. That's how Joseph from Cyprus, one of the assistant clergy at the worship center, got his new name. The leaders called him, "Cheery", because he sold his field and gave them the money. (2Luke 4: 32)

Saul made for Jerusalem and tried to join the followers of Jesus there. But they were all afraid of him and thought it was a trick. It was Cheery who befriended him and introduced him to those in charge. Cheery told them how Saul had met the Leader on the road, and how the Leader had spoken to him. He also told them about Saul's courage in speaking for Jesus in Damascus. Saul got to know the friends of Jesus well, and went all over Jerusalem speaking on behalf of the Leader. (9:26)

Joseph, nicknamed by the early Christians 'Cheery', was a native of Cyprus. He was also a 'Levite', a member of the tribe of Israel which had special duties in the Temple. This means that, like Paul, Cheery drew on experience both from the very centre of Jewish religious life, and from the circumference. In Cyprus Cheery was brought up surrounded by those whose culture and religion was not Jewish, as was Paul in Tarsus. For both Paul and Cheery, this meant they were more than averagely proficient not only in their own Hebrew and Aramaic languages, but also in Greek, and probably, in the case of Paul at least, Latin. However hard we try, we can never block out entirely the influences that have contributed to our personalities, especially not those from our earliest days. It looks as if Paul (when he was still 'Saul') tried hard to do so, but failed. Later he admitted his indebtedness to both Jews and Gentiles, giving him the facility to be "all things to all people." But in the case of Joseph from Cyprus the mix was more constructive at an earlier stage. Joseph stepped easily and comfortably from his privileged position as a member of a lower order of the Jewish clergy into being a hearty member of 'The Way', as the followers of Jesus were called before they were called Christians. He was not called 'Cheery' for nothing. ('Son of Encouragement' is far too stilted a translation of Barnabas!) To get this nickname he must have been bubbling over. He showed his generous nature by selling a plot of land and giving the money to the Jesus community. Presumably the land was somewhere near Jerusalem, though we are not told exactly where it was. It might even have been back home in Cyprus. More likely the plot was a fringe benefit he received as a Levite, some land to build a house for his retirement, perhaps, or even more likely, somewhere to build a tomb for himself and his family. We do not know precisely what a Levite's duties in the Worship Centre were in the days of Jesus, but it seems Levites were not unlike today's Cathedral vergers. They looked after the fabric, acted as guides to the visitors, assisted in the slaughtering of the animals, and sang in the choir. They would have received generous helpings from the outrageous temple exchange rates, the sale of animals and temple souvenirs, as well as numerous special offerings known as 'tithes'. They were not supposed to engage in manual work, either on the land or in industry. So, perhaps not by today's standards, and someway short of the luxury enjoyed by Guy (Caiaphas) the Chief of the Clergy, by the standards of the day they would have been thought privileged and comfortable. Cheery was perhaps like those wealthy people who opt to support the Labour Party in solidarity with the less well off.

Cheery was relaxed and bright spirited, but none the less high principled. He did not, like many others, reject or fear a man with the reputation of being a bigot and a bully. He saw through to the sensitive nature Saul tried so hard to hide, saw the struggle and the pain, and recognized Saul's potential. Cheery was someone who, enjoying the confidence and respect of others, was well placed to perform the role of introducing the awkward and shy new-comer. Cheery stood by Saul after Saul's conversion and dipping in Damascus and introduced him to the leaders of the Jesus community in Jerusalem. Together Cheery and Paul became a missionary team, appointed by the multi-cultured, multi-colored fellowship of Antioch in Syria, to the task of taking the Good News to Cyprus. Cheery's first hand knowledge of the island, its culture, politics and possibilities, must have been invaluable, and his humanity and common sense a foil for Saul's impatient enthusiasm. As we have seen, Cheery was to show the same spirit in standing up for his nephew John Mark, when, in Paul's opinion, the young man had failed the test of loyalty. Cheery's faith in Mark, as previously his faith in Paul, proved to be well founded, and eventually Paul was to agree. Cheery and Mark built on the initial success of the mission to Cyprus. How long their work there together lasted we do not know. Perhaps for Cheery it was his life-long assignment. We know that Mark later travelled to Rome and joined Paul's team, as well as being the author of the first of the four great accounts of the ministry of Jesus. Cheery, for his part, wrote a letter that has survived and was widely accepted as authentic in the early Church, but is not as useful for us as the letters of Paul. It was directed to some minority conservative Jewish Christian groups, and the matters dealt with are not those that concern us today. On the limited evidence we have, Paul was more gifted than Cheery at writing letters, whereas Cheery more gifted at handling people. However, the tone of authority that marks Cheery's letter, very similar to that of Paul, suggests that like Paul he regarded himself as an apostle. At the meeting of 'the apostles' in Jerusalem to discuss the Gentile question (2Luke 15), Paul and Cheery are obviously regarded as having the same standing as Rocky and James the brother of Jesus. No other apostles are mentioned by name. Luke calls Cheery and Paul apostles in 14:14, and both on that occasion and at the Jerusalem meeting, Cheery's name is placed before that of Paul. He was, after all, Paul's senior in the faith.

If Cheery was generally recognized as an apostle, not just by Luke, then we must regard it as more likely than not that Cheery had a first hand experience of the Resurrection of Jesus. Maybe when Paul came to write his first letter to the Christians at Corinth, Cheery was one of those Paul talks about as having witnessed the raised Jesus, but who had 'gone to their rest'. One thing we can be certain about is that if Cheery had been on duty in the temple during the time of Jesus, he could not have missed the great teacher. Jesus frequently taught in the temple and his sessions were very popular. The Levites were also trained teachers in the scriptures and would have listened in as part of what they were called to do. The demonstration led by Jesus against the misuse of the temple precincts as trading areas would have had special significance for the Levites. They were mentioned in the prophesies relating to God's Chosen (Messiah).

The Lord whom you seek will suddenly come to his temple…
and he will purify the descendants of Levi…
until they present offerings to the Lord in righteousness.
(Malachi 3.NRSV)

For Cheery the event would have an extra dimension, for Jesus was also protesting against the exclusion of the Gentiles, and Cheery, although a Jew, came from a Gentile land and probably had Gentile friends. 'Offerings in righteousness' for Cheery as well as Jesus might well have meant a spiritual alternative to the slaughter of animals, an idea expressed by many of the prophets in the Hebrew scriptures. Perhaps the kind and gentle 'Cheery' was fed up with his job! If he was in those days the same likeable and helpful person as later described by Luke, then he would have been popular and a leader among his fellow Levites. It is likely, therefore, that when he moved from being a temple Levite to become a prominent follower of Jesus, he took some other Levites with him. Cheery is part of the substantial evidence that not all the Jewish clergy were against Jesus. Some were rabidly opposed to him; others were not sure; and some moved slowly but surely to Jesus' side. The Letter of Barnabas was possibly written to some of his old mates.

For Luke, however, there was no doubt. Cheery was an apostle. And that was not because he threw his authoritative weight about, like Rocky and Paul, but because, in modest tones, he gave wise counsel and encouragement where sorely needed, and because he played a leading role in taking the Good News to his own land.

John Mark

Harry sends his best wishes. He's in prison too. Mark (Cheery's cousin), also sends his greetings. (I've already asked you to give a warm welcome to Mark, if ever he visits you.) Justin sends his kind regards. These are the only Jewish Christians here willing to work with me to bring about God's New World. They've been a tremendous help!...

My very good friend, Dr. Luke, and Demas, send their greetings.....

I, PAUL, AM TAKING OVER THE PEN TO WRITE THIS BIT OF THE LETTER MYSELF. PLEASE REMEMBER ME WHILE I'M IN PRISON. MAY YOU KNOW GOD'S GOODNESS AND LOVE.(Letter from Paul and his team to Quaketown [Colossians chapter 4.])

Only Luke is with me. Get Mark and bring him with you, because he can help me in the work.(From the unauthentic '2nd Letter of Paul to Timothy. 4:11. However, the greetings and personal asides in the letter are thought by many scholars to have been culled from genuine letters of Paul.)

For a full reconstruction of the career of John Mark, imaginative but securely based on the scriptures, I must direct my readers to my book *'The Gay Disciple'*. I believe that much of Mark's knowledge of Jesus was first hand, though he was a youngster at the time. He must also have, at a later date, collected stories from those who had had special encounters with Jesus in Galilee, including some from Jesus' inner circle, especially Rocky, if the tradition that Rocky was a prime source is to be trusted. Some of Mark's account of the Good News is obviously autobiographical. Mark puts himself into the story anonymously, as was the custom for a narrator. Luke does not mention his own name in his two-volume work, but refers to himself in the 'we passages'. Larry, Jesus' special friend, whose memory was responsible for much of 'Sources Close', including the last chapter (trad. 'John's Gospel'), used the pseudonym 'the disciple Jesus loved'. (Whoever put the whole gospel together made the identity unambiguously clear in chapter eleven.) It was probably Mark's parents' large house, maybe a hotel, that was the scene of 'The Last Supper', and the receiving of God's Spirit at Pentecost. It continued, almost certainly, to be one of the main meeting points for Christians in Jerusalem, and was where Rocky went for refuge after escaping from prison. The first Christians popped in and out of one another's' homes in the same way as people did in the valleys of Wales in my youth, but whereas the end of the coal industry and its close community has largely put paid to the practice in Wales, it was persecution that put paid to it in Jerusalem. Mark and his family, like most of the other Christian families, fled the city for places like Jaffa, Damascus and Antioch in the north. Rocky turns up at lodgings in Jaffa, and John Mark and his uncle Cheery are to be found at Antioch where they team up with Saul (Paul). This took Mark through Galilee, and he may have picked up some of his stories as he fled, hiding in the house of one Jesus sympathiser after another. Whatever the bone of contention between Paul and Mark, in which Cheery took Mark's side, Luke does not go into details. But Luke does suggest that it was Paul who was being difficult, and Cheery's established affability must also be put into the balance against Paul. Despite his youth (and he was getting older) Mark was a man of character and spirit, as his reminiscences of the last days of Jesus on earth demonstrate.

We do not know how long Mark and Cheery stayed on Cyprus during their second visit without Paul, but Mark did not end his days there. He turns up at Rome as one of Paul's team, as Paul's letters attest. Not only does Paul value Mark as a companion, but also a trusted stand-in to visit the churches on his behalf. This means that at sometime Paul and Mark were reconciled. It must have been a touching scene. We would like to think this meant that Paul came to appreciate Mark's qualities and the special knowledge of Jesus he held, both as an eye-witness to the events of the Passion and Resurrection, and as a collector of information from the stories of others. He had become one of Paul's deputies, a deputy-apostle or more likely an apostle in his own right. The fact that his name was regarded as carrying sufficient authority to be attached to the name of his gospel, attests his apostleship. Two of the gospels (Matthew and John) resort to using the name of a more prominent apostle, because the name of the actual author carried insufficient weight. If we had to choose between the loss of Apostle Mark's gospel and the letters of Apostle Paul, what would our choice would be, I wonder? A good topic for a University degree question!

Silas

Then the whole meeting agreed to choose representatives to send to Antioch with Paul and Cheery. The two they chose were respected leaders of the Christian community, Jude and Silas. The letter they took with them read like this:

This letter is to those from a non-Jewish background who trust in Jesus, in Antioch and the surrounding districts. It comes to you from the leaders of the Christian community and friends of Jesus in Jerusalem. We are sorry to hear that some people from our number visited you and, without our backing, said things to upset you and cause trouble. The representatives we are sending you have the support of all of us. They will travel alongside our much loved Cheery and Paul, who have risked their lives in the cause of Jesus, our Leader. Our representatives are Jude and Silas. They will explain the contents of this letter to you.... (2Luke 15)

This is a letter from Paul, Silas and Timothy, to the Christian community in Tessatown. We're writing on behalf of The Loving God and The Leader, Jesus, God's Chosen. It comes with our best wishes and concern for your happiness.

(Letters from Paul's Team – First Letter to Tessatown)

We know very little about Silas except that he was an important figure among the first Christians. Like Paul, he was both Jewish and a Roman citizen, and probably a competent linguist with Latin, Hebrew, Greek and Aramaic. He was therefore highly intelligent, literate and cultured. We do not know whether, like Paul, he was or had been a Pharisee. More likely he was a 'scribe', that is 'an expert in the old books'. These are frequently lumped together with the Pharisees, but were in fact a distinct group, sometimes overlapping, sometimes not. Like Paul, Silas was able to relate to the thought patterns of both Jew and Gentile, but unlike Paul he seems to have been an ideal arbitrator, adept at handling people. He was chosen for such a task by the meeting of leaders traditionally known as 'The Council of Jerusalem' as if it were the very first of the Church's official 'Councils', which it probably was not. It was crucially important none the less. The subject was the admission of Gentiles, as Gentiles, into the Christian community, and what was to be required of them. Silas was without doubt a member of that meeting, which came to a very wise and momentous decision. However, the task of explaining the provisions of the resultant 'apostolic' letter to the Christians of Antioch, the hub of Gentile Christianity at the time, was not entrusted to the big guns Paul and Cheery alone. We may imagine that this was because Paul was thought to be too quick tempered, and Cheery, at the other end of the scale, too laid back. Besides, both were biased towards the Gentile cause. Jude and Silas were just right. There were lots of Judes about in the early Church and it is not possible to say whether this Jude was one of the Judes we meet in the gospel lists of apostles or as the 'Judas not the one from Kerioth' in 'Sources Close'. It seems likely, though, that both were residents of Jerusalem, and that means possible witnesses of Jesus' execution and rising. Neither were in the original lists of apostles, but since the other apostles were becoming scarcer by the day, Jude and Silas may already have achieved the status of stand-ins.

When Paul had his sharp disagreement with Cheery and the two decided to go separate ways, it was Silas who agreed to become Paul's new sidekick. The fact that he agreed to accept this role must tell us something about Silas' character. Paul's tiff with Cheery and his unwillingness to forgive Mark only confirmed the already established general view that Paul was a difficult customer and not easy to get on with. Silas felt sufficiently confident to have a go, and although it is 'Paul and Silas' nearly all the way (not 'Silas and Paul'), nevertheless, in the stories Luke recounts, we can feel Silas' strong and calm presence as an essential factor in keeping the show on the road. (Silas was one of those natural seconds-in-command, without whom number one would find it difficult to operate. (Notice also: Judas and Silas, not Silas and Jude!)) Paul hated being on his own, as both his letters and Luke's account of him show over and over. At the same time he was not easy to live with, and his friends had to be very special and very understanding. At Lester (Lystra) Paul made a new friend in Timothy, and there has been much speculation about the strength and nature of Paul's feelings for this younger man (as in the novel of my good friend the late Vesper Hunter, 'Beloved Brother'.) The team was now to be 'Paul, Silas and Timothy' and as we may have experienced ourselves, 'two is company and three a crowd'. There is no evidence of any tension, and with somebody like Silas we would not expect very much. Luke made up a foursome from time to time, and that would have helped. Paul, Silas and Timothy were still together when Paul wrote some of his earliest surviving letters, the two letters to Tessatown. These letters are not from Paul, but from 'Paul, Silas and Timothy'. The first letter shows the memory of the group's first strike missionary activity in Macedonia and Greece, including the spot of bother in Philiptown. It also expresses the anxiety of Paul for his converts to behave responsibly in sexual matters, which may reveal something of his anxieties about himself. Many scholars believe that at this time Silas, using the Latin version of his name, Silvanus, acted as Paul's scribe, since Paul had a problem with his eyes and could only read and write large print. We cannot tell how much of the letter is Paul or how much Silas or Timothy for that matter, but Paul sometimes intervenes to say 'PAUL SPEAKING NOW', proof the others definitely had a hand. Silas drops out of the later letters of Paul and it is just 'from Paul and Timothy'. So perhaps eventually the threesome did become a bit of a strain. Silas seems later to have joined Rocky in Rome as his scribe for his letter-cum-Easter sermon, 'The call to Hope.' Mark was also there at the time, no doubt making notes for his gospel. Silas would have been just as interesting a source as Rocky, being able to help Mark with some of the Jerusalem background, especially if he had knowledge of what went on in the council that put Jesus on trial. In the Christian scriptures from that time it is Rocky who has the last word on Silas. It agrees with the rest of our limited but consistent knowledge of him.

*Silas has been helping me write all this down. **He's a reliable friend**. I hope my words will encourage you and that you'll realize they bear the true mark of God. Keep a tight grip on reality! Your Christian friends in the big city send their kind regards.Mark also sends his greetings. He's a like a son to me. Give one another a big kiss every time you meet! I send my own best wishes for the peace and happiness of all of you who are friends of Jesus.*

'The Call to Hope' (1 Peter) chapter 5.

Chapter Seventeen

Luke's Apostles (Continued 2)

Lydia

The boat from Troy took us straight across the Aegean Sea and next day up the coast to Newtown. After we had landed, we made for Philiptown, the largest town in those parts. The population is largely Italian. We spent a few days getting to know the place. Then on Saturday we went down by the river outside the town, where we heard people were in the habit of meeting to talk with God. It turned out to be a women's group, so we sat and chatted to those who had come along. One of them, Lydia, was a business woman, who owned a company that made high quality purple cloth. God was already important in her life, so she listened very carefully to everything Paul said, and took it all in. Lydia, and the people who lived with her, were dipped in the river. Then she invited us back to her house. She said. "Now I've put my trust in Jesus, you're welcome to come and stay with me." So we went home with her. (2Luke 16: 11-15)

I can't tell you how much I miss you, dear friends. You're my prize converts, and just thinking about you makes me happy. I love you very much. Stay loyal to the Leader.

It's time for Edna and Cynthia to put an end to their disagreement. That's what the Leader wants. I'm asking Lydia, the one who worked with me to establish your community, and who has my trust, to give them some support. They all worked hard with me in spreading the good news. So did Clem, and the others in the team. God has made a note of their names. (Letter to Philiptown chapter 4).

The 'We' passages, in which Luke indicates that he has now become involved in events, begin at the point where the Good News is to be taken over the water from Asia to Europe. Luke has

181

often been identified with 'The Man from Macedonia' who Paul encountered in a dream, calling "Come over to Macedonia and help us!" The scenario is this: Paul, accompanied by Silas and Timothy were making their way through central 'Asia Minor', Turkey as it now is. They were 'prevented by the Spirit' every time they tried to enter a town or community for the purposes of evangelism. Maybe Paul was experiencing one of his frequent bouts of sickness, something like epilepsy perhaps, or at any rate something leading to physical loss of energy with accompanying problems of vision. The thesis continues on the lines that the group were obliged to make for the far western coast where the weather would be more moderate and the sea air do Paul good. There he met Dr. Luke who attended to his illness, perhaps by having a good bedside chat with Paul about his mission and suggesting that the peoples of Macedonia and Greece were in dire need of what Paul had to offer. So, during the night, Paul had his dream of the 'Man from Macedonia', looking a bit like Dr. Luke through the dreamy haze. In the morning, Paul interpreted his dream as guidance and the group, now with Luke as Paul's personal physician, set sail from Troy to Newtown Macedonia, the very next day. Thence they proceeded to Philiptown, the nearest large town, and a Roman colony. Though there was trouble in store, it was to prove one of the most successful visits of Paul's team to any town. A thriving, well-ordered, and happy church was the result, proving beyond doubt the authenticity of the vision. That's the story-line and it makes sense. We must now add to the story the big surprise, not often noted by male-fixated commentators of times past. The 'Man from Macedonia' turned out to be a woman! Well, dreams *are* hazy!

Paul's usual plan of action when entering a new town was to look for the synagogue, the Jewish place of worship. But Philiptown was a thoroughly Gentile town, and did not possess among its inhabitants even the required twelve Jewish men to enable a synagogue to function. What was Paul to do now? He was stumped until he learned that there was a group that met every Saturday by the river for prayer. Having not very much information, perhaps, Paul would have been surprised to find that he was going to have to make do for his Sabbath worship with a women's group, maybe not Jewish, but earnest and sincere and above all seeking God. There are many such groups outside the walls of our churches today, engaging in many types of what is described by the umbrella word 'spirituality'. We mistrust them, since, not being under our direction, their theologies or lack of them are unlikely to be 'sound', even to the more liberal of us. I recently attended by accident a retreat organized by those who still practice the religion of the ancient Celts of these islands. I had booked in for another retreat, but since that retreat did not have suitable accommodation for me, I simply transferred my deposit to the group meeting the following week. I had a very interesting time, and found much in common with the other retreaters, though I'm sure many of my colleagues would have been horrified. I returned home the possessor of a genuine magic wand. It is still in my study and I have not used it yet! I wonder, when Paul saw the little group of women worshipping at the river, where in ancient times nature gods and river sprites were to be found, he might have been tempted to turn back. He was not too keen on women either – not perhaps a misogynist, as is sometimes asserted, but certainly uneasy in the company of women, as the Pharisees were in general. Members of the 'Strict Set' would look away at the approach of a woman unknown to them, which explains the words of Jesus, intended as tongue-in-cheek, "If your eye offends you, pluck it out!" Paul might have wondered whether he would be welcome. Religious men frequently excluded women from their meetings. These women might not welcome men into their midst. Lydia was their leader. She welcomed Paul, Silas and Timothy and made them feel at ease. She had an open mind and heart to new ideas and she and her friends were convinced of the truth of Paul's message. They responded by being dipped there and then in the river. These women were seekers and now they had found what they had been looking for. Why delay? What a contrast they make to the average Christian when presented with something new and different. What a contrast to the response Paul usually got in the synagogue, more often than not carping and critical. But Lydia was no ordinary woman.

Lydia was a business woman. Her business was selling purple cloth, the most expensive and sought after fabric, used for the Emperor's clothing and for that of his closest attendants or members of the royal family. Lydia probably inherited the firm from her father, or from her husband and must have been very wealthy. Her house would have been a grand one, a villa on the Roman style most likely, with a large household of servants and slaves. To run such a company required both business skills and overall intelligence, as well as ability in handling employees. Whatever Paul's feelings about women being in charge of things, he knew immediately that in Lydia he had found a gem. Paul was quite capable of making exceptions to his prejudices when it suited him. Without doubt Lydia fitted naturally into the role of leader of the new Christian community in Philiptown. She was highly respected in the town, if only for her business skills and ability to organize people. The mission of the early Christian Church did not involve erecting church buildings. If Paul found he could not use the already existing synagogues, he would hire a lecture hall, or use a Greek amphitheatre, or in the case of Philiptown, the riverside. Then new converts would meet in the houses of the more wealthy among their number, where there would be good catering and toilet facilities. A villa was a town, or a 'village' in itself, and with the influx of new converts, would have been a very busy place indeed. There is a discernible theme running through the brief account of Paul's 'conversion' of Lydia. My father had a sermon about it, in which he used the old 3-point plan. Lydia, he told his congregation, 1) opened her heart 2) opened her home and 3) made an 'open confession'. The third point was his opportunity as a typical Baptist of his day to give the invitation to 'Believers' Baptism'. Despite the seeming simplicity of the plan and each of the three points, we were given the ideal picture of a seeker after God and God's truth. Lydia possessed the kind of mind that was open to receive new ideas and explore new pathways, at the same time unhesitating at the point when a vital decision was required. She was also prepared to stand up and be counted, openly and publicly, despite the consequences. One of these consequences must have been the disruption, to the point of chaos at times, of her well ordered and happy home. I have a strong feeling that one of the reasons Christians of later times were so keen on erecting church buildings, great and small, was to discourage unwanted visitors from arriving at their homes. Hospitality was a basic feature of early Christianity. Those who owned the bigger houses opened them up. It was not in the spirit of Jesus to be choosy, though some tried, as the letter of James shows. We do not get the true picture unless we realise that it is not a church building that James is talking about, but somebody's home.

If you pay special attention to the one who's well-dressed and say, "Please take a seat" and then say to the one who looks down and out, "Stand over there" or "You can sit on the floor", you're being snobbish and judging on the basis of prejudice.

(The Call to Action Chapter 2.)

It's all very well to say things like that, James, and you are, of course, quite right. It is not so simple in practice. Asking a Roman senator's wife to sit on the floor and giving the most comfortable seat to someone who looked and smelt as if a bath was long overdue, must have been a tricky exercise. My room in college was a meeting point at 10.30 pm for those wishing a cup of cocoa or *Ovaltine* with a pleasant chat or some classical music before going to bed. It was not uncommon for one member of the student body to come in and another to get up straight away and walk out. In our small confined community there were those who did not like one another and the best way of preserving peace, though perhaps not the most Christian way, was strategic avoidance. Among the Christians of Philiptown meeting at Lydia's place, were Edna and Cynthia (Euodia and Syntache) who could not stand the sight of each another, and after five minutes in the same room were at each other's throats. Paul urges Lydia to deal with the problem, for they are poisoning the whole atmosphere of the community. According to the Greek manuscripts we have received Paul does not mention Lydia by name. This looks like one of several places in the scriptures where copyists removed the names of women when they wished to bury the evidence that women had places of leadership in the early Church. It is a rather obvious omission since Clement, the other well-known leader (the prison governor most likely), is mentioned by name, and also the two women miscreants – alright to name women who served as examples of women as a disruptive influence. It is almost unbelievable that Paul would not name Lydia, for not to do so would be ungracious. He calls her his 'partner'. The Greek is 'sunzugos', which means 'somebody yoked together with me'. It signifies an equal, because if oxen were unequally yoked, both would stumble. Paul is calling to mind, many years later, how he and Lydia together, working in partnership, had established the church at Philiptown, and he appeals to her, knowing her relia-bility and impartiality, to do something about these fractious women. It makes more sense if it is a woman, a Christian 'sister', who is being asked to do this. Whether or not the early Christians regarded Lydia as an 'apostle', she was recognized as being among the prominent leaders of the Church, and Paul who awarded himself the title, regarded Lydia as his equal. The title you give someone does not really matter. It's doing the job that counts.

Off on a tangent, it would be interesting to know what happened to the mystic 'Pythoness' who Paul converted in Philiptown, between the conversions of Lydia and Clement. This is arguably the story of another of Paul's bad acts, since this woman would not have ended up a Christian had she not pestered Paul to the point of action, like the woman with a law suit in Jesus' parable. The early Christians seem to have been thrown as to what to do about members of the magic circle who were attracted to the cause. This young witch was a 'clairvoyant' who used a python as a ventriloquist's mouthpiece to deliver her predictions. It is impossible to know whether a clairvoyant's predictions in a particular case result from genuine psychic insight, or from guesswork. Be that as it may, the Pythoness identified Paul and Silas accurately as men of God and followed them around pointing them out to everybody. This annoyed Paul, unreasonably, since she was heartily recommending Paul's mission to the citizens of Philiptown. At last Paul 'cured' her of her psychic abilities, rendering her useless to her employers, who then had Paul and Silas arrested. Presumably this woman, whose name might also have been removed from the text by a copyist, joined the church in Lydia's villa. Was her name Edna (Euodia)? Or Cynthia (Syntache)? Or Romana? Did she regain her psychic powers and become a prophetess within the fellowship, or did she suffer frustration at the loss of her special gift? Was she a valued member of the group, or one of those doggedly loyal attendees who has to be endured with Christian patience? We hope Lydia managed to sort her out!

Ray (Apollos)

Meanwhile, in Ephesus, a Jew from northern Africa called Ray arrived. He was a good speaker and knew the old books well. He had been instructed in the basic truths of Christianity, and was very keen to pass on what he had learnt. His knowledge of the facts about Jesus was very accurate. He seemed, however, not to know about any dipping of people

since the time of John the Dipper. He courageously spoke his mind in the worship place. Cill and Will were among those who heard Ray. They invited him home, and explained to him aspects of Christianity he had not come across. Ray wanted to visit Greece. So the Christians of Ephesus made things easier for him by writing letters of introduction to the Greek Christians. When Ray arrived in Greece, he was a great help to those Greeks who had accepted God's gift. He entered into public debate with the Jewish leaders, and was able to show, by using the old books, that Jesus is God's Chosen.
   2Luke 18:24.

*Those rival fan clubs of yours,- "I'm in Paul's gang!" or "I'm in Ray's gang!",- just show how immature you are! What's so big about Ray or Paul? We're only helpers, doing the job God has given us. I put the plants in their pots, and Ray came along with the watering can. It was God who got the plants to grow*1Corinthians 3:4

There is no way we can avoid the conclusion that the scriptures we possess are a very unbalanced account of what actually happened historically. Whether they are also unbalanced from a theological point of view will depend very much on one's theology. The two are almost certainly connected. We know more about Paul than almost anyone else, including Jesus, more than we know about the 'twelve' apostles apart from Rocky, more than we know about Jesus' family, including his mother, more than we know about Joseph from Ram and Nick, more than we know about Maggie (Mary Magdala – 'Mary the Magnificent'), and countless others who can be seen from the gospels to have played a leading role in the early Christian communities. The common assumption is that it was the work of Paul that got the Church going, especially outside the Holy Land, as if, had there been no Paul, primitive Christianity would have petered out. I have heard this stated many times on television programs as if it were historical fact. The fact is that Paul had an accomplished biographer and the others did not. It is like saying there would have been no abolition of the slave trade if there had been no William Wilberforce. It might have happened later without Wilberforce, but it would have happened. Luke's opinion of Paul was not Paul's opinion of himself. False modesty, perhaps, but Paul looked upon himself as 'the least'. Apart from the mission team led by this ebullient and energetic man (though often inactive due to exhaustion), there were many other individuals and teams taking the Good News not only westwards to Greece and Rome, but southwards to Africa and eastwards to Persia and India. And this was not because it was Paul's big idea, but because it was what Jesus had told his friends he wanted them to do. Although Rocky and Co. were slow off the mark, others were not. Despite his big build up of Paul's work, Luke was aware of the contribution made by others. We just wish he had told us more.

Ray is what we call Apollos in 'Good As New', for his name is that of the Greek sun god. Luke tells us he was a native of Alexandria and therefore geographically African. But culturally he was most probably a member of the sizeable Jewish colony in that city. The Alexandrian Jews were Greek speaking and much influenced by Greek culture. However it is not impossible that Apollos was an Egyptian, a Jew by conversion rather than race. Many Jews had Greek names, but 'Apollos' is more pagan than most. His local name may have been 'Aten', the name of the Egyptian sun god, which became Apollos when translated into Greek. We have gone one step further and translated it into English. Be that as it may, there is no doubt that Ray was a scholar, a highly regarded teacher, and a scholar/teacher who kept abreast of the very latest ideas, including those of Jesus of Nazareth. Ray had researched the life and teaching of Jesus and as a result became a Jesus person. That does not preclude the possibility that he had also seen, met or heard Jesus teach on a visit to Jerusalem for one of the festivals. Jesus liked to be at the festivals in order to meet the pilgrims from other countries.

Apollos had learnt that Jesus had about twelve disciples to help him with his mission, so Apollos took a team of approximately that number with him to spread the Good News. Ray's team and Paul's team seem to have first become aware of the other's existence when Ray reached Ephesus. Paul was, at that time, evangelizing the nearby Celtic lands. Paul had left Ephesus in the capable hands of the married couple Cill and Will. The time sequence is not quite clear and it may be that Ray arrived before Cill and Will and had already started his Ephesus mission. Some scholars think it is to Ray rather than Paul that the foundation of the Church at Ephesus is to be attributed. It must have been quite a surprise to Cill and Will to find a complete stranger preaching in the synagogue, eloquently extolling the merits of Jesus, just like Paul. It was not surprising that Ray had a different take on Jesus from that of Cill and Will whose thinking had been influenced by Paul. With respect to baptism, Ray had only heard about John the Dipper. This does not necessarily mean that Ray had only heard about 'baptism for repentance'. More likely it means, since Ray's interest was in Jesus, that all he knew about dipping was John's dipping of Jesus. He had not heard about the events of the Day of Pentecost and the mass dippings on that occasion, or the continuing of the practice as an initiation ceremony in the Christian community.

The impression we get is that Ray thanked Cill and Will for putting him right and that thereafter he included an invitation to be dipped in the name of Jesus in his sermons. But there may be more to it. The appearance of Ray on the scene, almost from nowhere, with a well-trained team, alerts us to the historical certainty that there were any number of Christian missions each with their own version of the Good News and with differing customs and expectations of what was called for from their converts. Some of these, as we know from Paul's letters, were vehemently opposed to Paul's version of Christianity and followed him about everywhere he went, causing him trouble. A close study of 'Sources Close' (John's Gospel) reveals another version of Jesus and his teaching from that of the other three gospels, also from that of Paul and from that of Paul's fundamentalist critics. Sources Close includes no mention of Jesus being dipped and has the statement that Jesus did not dip. It was his disciples who did the dipping. 'Sources Close' also says that the Holy Spirit was given by Jesus personally at Eastertime rather than to the waiting Church at Pentecost. Ray may have shown deference and humility in his acceptance of Cill and Will's way of understanding things, but maybe he was right or at least entitled to his own alternative. Maybe Jesus would have preferred dipping as an option rather than an imposition. Even Paul said, "Jesus didn't ask me to dip people. He asked me to pass on the Good News."(1Corinthians: 1:16)We can see already the way the Church is going to go, confusing uniformity in the matter of non-essentials with the unity that comes from allegiance to Jesus before all else.

At all events, Ray does not become a rival of Paul's, but an ally. He has his own outfit; he does not merge with Paul; we do not even know whether he and Paul ever actually met, though quite likely they did. They took care not to tread on each other's toes. At the point where Paul seemed likely to return to Ephesus, Ray set sail for Corinth with letters of introduction from Cill and Will. In Corinth Ray built on the work of Paul, and drew words of appreciation from Paul in his first letter to the community there.

'I put the plants in their pots, and Ray came along with the watering can.' (1Corinthians 3)

It is very obvious in that letter that Paul regards Ray as being an equal with himself and with Rocky. The Corinthians had divided themselves into fan clubs based on their favorite teachers, but none of the leaders would approve of the use of their names in this way. In the opinion of Paul, at any rate, Ray merited the title 'apostle'. Luke does not seem to have had much chance to assess Ray's work or have knowledge of his subsequent career, but he would have accepted Paul's assessment of him. Ray was one of the key figures in the early Church, and that is why I would pass him over as a possible author of 'The Call to Trust' ('Hebrews'). There would have been no problem in preserving the letter under the name of 'Apollos'. His name would have carried sufficient weight for it to be regarded as 'apostolic'. Whereas The Letter to the Hebrews took some time to become established. Read on.

Cill and Will.

Paul went on from Athens to Corinth. There he met a Jewish couple, Cilla and William, who came originally from the Black Sea coast. They had recently moved to Corinth from Rome because the Emperor Claudius had turned all the Jews out of Rome. Paul went to see them and they took him in as a lodger. They got on well because they were all skilled tentmakers. They set up business together. 2Luke 18

Give my kind regards to Cill and Will, my Christian workmates. They gave their lives for me. I'm grateful to them, and so are all our groups. My regards to the Christians who meet in their house.

Paul's Letter to Rome 16:3.

Will and Cill, and the Christian group which meets in their house, send their warmest greetings.. 1Corinth 16:19.

Sarah, Abraham's wife, was able to have a baby, even though she was past the normal age of having children. That was because she trusted God to keep a promise.

When he (Moses) became an adult, he gave up his privileges as the adopted son of Pharaoh's daughter.

Barbara (Rahab) was a prostitute whose trust was rewarded. She entertained spies from the Jewish camp and so didn't die with those who had not sided with God.

Women who thought their children dead had them back again, alive and well Extracts 'The Call to Trust (Hebrews) chapter 11.

The last apostle for our imagined list of Luke's alternative apostles is an apostle with two heads, or rather two bodies, which cannot be thought of without the other. Cill and Will were a husband and wife team. Sometimes in the manuscripts, which do not always agree, it is 'Priscilla (or Prisca) and Aquila', sometimes 'Aquila and Priscilla'. Some scholars, Harnack for example, believe the manuscripts that put Aquila first have been tampered with to ensure male priority. But even when we use the translations in which the couple take turns to be mentioned first, it should be noted that Luke, introducing the couple for the first time, puts Will first, whereas when Luke records the two being charged by Paul with responsibility for the mission in Ephesus, he puts Cill first. This is so much against the ethos of the time that we must conclude that Cill led the duo rather than Will. We are told that Will came from the Black Sea coast, from a region of the ancient Asia Minor, whereas tradition has it that Cill was a native of Rome and a member of an aristocratic family. Both have Latin names, and both were of the Jewish faith before they became Christians. They were in the tent-making or leather trade, as was Paul. Maybe it was the combination of Cill's money and business acumen together with Will's skill as a craftsman that accounted for their firm's success. Like Lydia, Cill and Will were sufficiently well-off to be able to afford a house large enough to accommodate meetings of the Christian community. They happened to be in Corinth when Paul arrived there because they had been expelled from Rome during a Jewish pogrom instigated by the Emperor Claudius. It is not clear whether they were converts of Paul, or by contact with the Christian community which had already been established in Rome, possibly by Christians among the military or the civil service, whose duties took them from one end of the empire to the other.

Cill was a highly connected, intelligent, and cultured woman, educated both in Latin and Greek language and culture and in the Jewish faith. The reason why she is regarded by many as the author of Hebrews (Good as New 'The Call to Trust') is because she has all the necessary qualifications to fit the bill and no other name so far proposed does so. We find a thorough knowledge of the Hebrew Bible combined with the most polished Greek in the Christian scriptures, rivaled only by that of Luke. The author also possesses a mastery of classical rhetoric and an acquaintance with Greek philosophy. The reason Hebrews lacks an author, named in the text, is just as obvious. The author was a woman. Her name was removed, and no one could think of a plausible name to replace her. Paul will not do. His Greek style, or rather that of his secretaries, is quite different, nowhere near Priscilla's excellence. It took a long time for Hebrews to be accepted in the canon, probably because those in the know suspected the truth. But the work has so much to say that is not said anywhere else, it could not be jettisoned. 'The Call to Trust' speaks not only to those who were uncertain whether to be Christians or Jews in the first century, but to all in every age and every faith who need to understand the choice between being a friend of God on the one hand and being 'religious' on the other.

'The Call to Trust' in places has the feel of a feminist manifesto. Cilla includes in her 'Roll Call of Faith' (chapter 11) women whom a male author would have been unlikely to mention, including Sarah and the prostitute Barbara. In the case of Sarah, Cilla rewrites the scriptures which portray Sarah as laughing when the messengers from God say that she will give birth to a child. Instead, Cilla includes Sarah as one famed for her faith. For some copyists this radical approach to scripture was more than they could take and they cut out the sentences praising Sarah. Thus they do not appear in all the manuscripts and some traditional translations also leave them out. It is time Christians put back Cilla's name in the title to her work. After all, few scholars believe that Matthew was written by Matthew or John by John, so why are they honored in this way, while a much more likely author is erased from memory?

Whenever people today are asked to name the 12 apostles, they nearly always begin with Matthew, Mark, Luke and John, only two of whom were in the official list. But they are not wrong to regard Mark and Luke as apostles. They were apostles of the pen. They played as great a part in spreading the Good News in the first century as did Rocky and Paul and the rest. Cill too deserves to be honored not only as an apostle of the pen, but as a Christian leader and evangelist of the first rank.

The other apostle who should be mentioned is Luke. Without Luke Paul may not have been able to cope sufficiently with his physical ailments to have continued much of his work. Luke was probably responsible for keeping Paul sane on many occasions. He was with Paul at critical moments to give him support. At the same time Luke continued his journal and collection of stories about Jesus. Without Luke we would have no 'Prodigal Son' or 'Good Samaritan'; no criminal at the cross asking Jesus a favor, nor the prayer 'Forgive them, loving God…'; nor valuable information about Mary, the mother of Jesus. Luke gives us portraits of the first heroes of the Church with great honesty, perception, loyalty and love. The one who reports Jesus' prayer of forgiveness on the cross also relates the good acts and the bad acts of Jesus' friends, confident that God's loving forgiveness will cover all. Well done, Dr. Luke; well done, Luke the Apostle!

About the Author

John Henson is a native of Cardiff and a son of the Manse. He graduated in history and theology at the universities of Southampton and Oxford (Regent's Park) respectively and was ordained to the Baptist ministry at Carmel Baptist Church, Pontypridd in 1964. He was responsible for a union between his own church and the United Reformed Church in 1969 (now St. David's, Pontypridd) and has since given assistance to other churches seeking to make similar unions at the local level. He taught history in Cardiff High School from 1970 - 1973 and then resumed ministry at Glyncoch, Pontypridd in cooperation with the Anglican Communion.

Since 1980 he has been largely freelance, acting as pastoral befriender to people in minority groups while continuing to assist in the conduct of worship in the churches. One has now folded up! interests include music, left-wing politics, penal reform, peace, the quest for truly contemporary and inclusive worship and gender issues. A member of the Lesbian and Gay Christian Movement from its early years, for many years he assisted the movement as the contact person for the South Wales group and as a counsellor. He has lectured on faith and gender in Strasbourg and Oslo at the invitation of the European Union and the World Student Christian Federation. He has also lectured in the U.K. at ecumenical conferences and retreat centres, and at Greenbelt. He is happily married to Valerie, his partner for forty-five years. They have three adult children, Gareth, Iestyn and Rhôda, and nine grandchildren-Aidan, Bleddyn, Carys, Gwenllian, Dyfrig, Iona, Isobel, Tomos and Ffion-Medi.

John Henson's books to date are the *'Other'* series *'Other Temptations of Jesus'*, *'Other Communions of Jesus'* and *'Other Prayers of Jesus'*; *"Good-As-New"- translation of the Christian scriptures*; and

'*The Gay Disciple*'. Still to come, '*Other Friends of Jesus*', '*Heaven and Hell – a dish of hot potatoes*', '*The Love Line- Scriptural understandings of Gender*', and the Welsh language version of *Good As New*'.

BOOKS

O is a symbol of the world, of oneness and unity. In different cultures it also means the "eye," symbolizing knowledge and insight. We aim to publish books that are accessible, constructive and that challenge accepted opinion, both that of academia and the "moral majority."

Our books are available in all good English language bookstores worldwide. If you don't see the book on the shelves ask the bookstore to order it for you, quoting the ISBN number and title. Alternatively you can order online (all major online retail sites carry our titles) or contact the distributor in the relevant country, listed on the copyright page.

See our website **www.o-books.net** for a full list of over 500 titles, growing by 100 a year.

And tune in to myspiritradio.com for our book review radio show, hosted by June-Elleni Laine, where you can listen to the authors discussing their books.

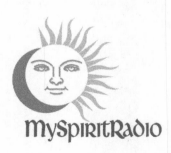

MySPIRITRADIO